The Medical Student Career Handbook

Edited by

Elizabeth Cottrell
Christele Rebora
Mark Williams
Foundation Year 1 Doctors

Foreword by

Steve Field

Radcliffe Publishing
Oxford • Seattle

Radcliffe Publishing Ltd
18 Marcham Road
Abingdon
Oxon OX14 1AA
United Kingdom

www.radcliffe-oxford.com
Electronic catalogue and worldwide online ordering facility.

British Library Cataloguing in Publication Data

A catalogue record for this book is available from the British Library.

ISBN-10 1 84619 077 0
ISBN-13 978 1 84619 077 3

Typeset by Advance Typesetting Ltd, Oxford
Printed and bound by TJ International Ltd, Padstow, Cornwall

A partnership between Keele University, the University of Warwick, the University of Birmingham and the West Midlands Deanery

UNIVERSITYOF
BIRMINGHAM

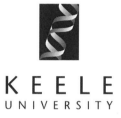

KEELE
UNIVERSITY

THE UNIVERSITY OF
WARWICK

WEST MIDLANDS
DEANERY

Contents

Foreword

I am delighted to write the foreword for this excellent book, whose arrival is timely given the introduction of new Foundation and Specialist Training Programmes across the United Kingdom.

The recent changes proposed in *Modernising Medical Careers* underline the importance of the benefits of informed career choice, not only in terms of efficient training programmes now, but also for the future generations of doctors. It is very likely that this will have added significance for those beginning a medical career later in life through the increasing number of UK based graduate entry programmes at medical school, or for medical graduates entering the NHS from Europe or from other parts of the world.

This book complements the UK wide approach to the delivery of career management initiatives that was launched as part of the Department of Health's *Modernising Medical Careers* strategy. As Chair of the working group that produced the national careers management strategy, I warmly welcome this book.

A key feature is that it has been researched and written by consumers; by final year medical students with contributions and support from more experienced consultants and general practitioners. I believe that it provides a superb source of information and focused help for medical students and junior doctors that will help them prepare effectively for their Foundation Programmes and for specialist training. It will also provide a valuable resource for educational supervisors, GP trainers and clinical tutors. I commend it to you.

Professor Steve Field
Postgraduate Dean, West Midlands
Chair, UK Modernising Medical Careers Advisory Board
July 2006

About the editors

All three editors were final-year medical students at Keele University when this *Handbook* was written.

Elizabeth Cottrell worked hard during her training to gain a broad knowledge and experience base. Her aim has always been to be a general practitioner (GP) but she is a firm believer in keeping career options open during medical school. As a result of this her work has been varied. In contrast to her time spent at a high-security forensic psychiatry hospital, she has assisted paediatric diabetes specialist nurses to gain funding for a nurse prescribing course and has been involved in laboratory research which has discovered some potentially exciting results. Elizabeth is currently in the process of setting up research on childhood diabetes and its management, with the aim of improving services to schools and teachers. She has experienced medicine from perspectives other than those of doctors, through nearly five years' part-time work as a healthcare assistant on orthopaedic and medical wards, a summariser of notes in a GP practice and as a hospital domestic earlier on in her career.

Christele Rebora has done a first degree in basic medical sciences. She initiated an ambassador-mentoring scheme for fourth-year medical students as part of the Widening Participation Scheme at Keele University. This scheme involves current medical students entering schools to promote higher education, university in general and medicine as a career; as well as providing advice and support about interviews and application procedures to those considering medicine. Christele is a great advocate of the importance of making an informed decision and of having the best and most accurate information in order to do this. Her work from previous projects includes compiling information used to train GP registrars, educating patients and formulating a checklist-learning tool for new doctors carrying out reports on children that may have special educational needs. She is also a volunteer with Heartstart, teaching cardiopulmonary resuscitation to members of the community, and has contributed to the 2007 Keele University Prospectus.

Mark Williams has previously been voted as the medical school's sports representative. In that position he encouraged other students to develop a work–life balance. Mark was also an active member of the Keele University Medical School student committee where he helped to raise funds for various medical student events and charities. Mark has been involved in work with a local youth forum, helping to organise music forum days allowing local children to develop constructive hobbies. Mark believes that medical students should increase their social conscience during medical school and learn how to balance work and social pressures.

About the contributors

Patrick Daly was a final-year student at Warwick University Medical School (WMS) when this *Handbook* was written. He graduated from Leicester University in 2002 after completing a BSc in medical biochemistry. Patrick moved the short distance down the M69 to Warwick to start the graduate entry course in medicine. He also founded the WMS Career Group and has organised several events for fellow students and hopes to continue this important role whilst working as a Foundation doctor in the local area.

Tracie Plant was a third-year student at Birmingham University Medical School when this *Handbook* was written and is the curriculum and welfare committee chair there. She intercalated in 2005 in BMedSci neuroscience and has previous experience as a course representative and welfare representative for Birmingham University medical students. Tracie's non-academic interests include playing rugby for the medics and a local team, and adventure runs.

Stephanie Triance was a final-year student at Warwick University Medical School (WMS) when this *Handbook* was written. After completing a BSc in physiology she spent a year working for a PR recruitment consultancy in London. She then spent several months travelling through South America before commencing the graduate entry course at Warwick. She and her colleagues have started a career focus group that aims to provide students with a cohesive career support network throughout their undergraduate medical training.

Naomi Tyrrell was a third-year student at Warwick University Medical School (WMS) when this *Handbook* was written. She is the WMS British Medical Association medical students' committee representative and also sits on the WMS intra-school committee. In the past Naomi has been the sports secretary for WMS MedSoc and was part of an initiative that taught basic life support in schools.

Other contributors

In addition to the content produced by the authors, other people have contributed significantly to this *Handbook*.

Charlene Binding is Career Management Associate at Trent Multi-Professional Deanery. Her role is to take forward the *Modernising Medical Careers* (MMC) career management agenda in the Trent region. She is a member of the newly formed national Medical Careers Advisers Network (MCAN) and the national MMC-subgroup for career management, which authored the Department of Health publication *Career Management: An Approach for Medical Schools, Deaneries, Royal Colleges and Trusts*.[1] Charlene's input to this *Handbook*, and her work with the Trent Multi-Professional Deanery is acknowledged with gratitude.

Ruth Chambers is the Director of Postgraduate General Practice education at the West Midlands Deanery and Professor of Primary Care at Staffordshire University. She has been a GP for 25 years and is the national education lead for the NHS Alliance. Some of Ruth's current initiatives include enthusing to others about supporting patients to practise self-care, enhancing GP recruitment and retention, and enabling health professionals' career development through effective career planning. Ruth has written a great deal for doctors and other health professionals, in more than 60 books, and she has enjoyed 'shadowing' Lizzie, Mark and Christele as they have written and organised this book.

Margaret Lawless is a senior human resources adviser and a recruitment consultant with experience in both large and small non-medical companies. Margaret's work, research and input into Chapter 20 proved invaluable.

Reference

1 Modernising Medical Careers Working Group for Careers Management. *Career Management: An Approach for Medical Schools, Deaneries, Royal Colleges and Trusts*. London: The Stationery Office, 2005.

Acknowledgements

As a result of the nature of the content of this *Handbook*, some content has been derived from key documents. Any use of other documents has been fully referenced.

First, we must sincerely thank Professor Steve Field, without whom this book would not have been possible. We would also like to thank Steve for writing the foreword and helping us to write those chapters relating to *Modernising Medical Careers*.

It is with thanks that we acknowledge that we are following in the footsteps of the work the Trent Multi-Professional Deanery have laid down with regards to career information for medical students. The Trent Multi-Professional Deanery and the University of Nottingham have produced a *Nottingham Medical School Career Handbook*.[1] Through recognising how worthwhile a document such as this is, we felt that a book containing such important information should be available to all medical students. We have welcomed the input and experience of Charlene Binding, who has assisted us with the development of this book.

We should like to sincerely thank all the people who participated in surveys which enabled us to compile the specialty profiles and experiences of others.

Thanks also to those people who approached and 'chased' doctors to help us obtain all the specialty profiles: Charlene Kennedy, a final-year medical student at Manchester University who has also studied at St Andrews and Keele University medical schools; Nathalie Rebora, a final-year medical student from St George's International Medical School; and Jenny Robertson, a final-year medical student from Newcastle upon Tyne University Medical School.

We should like to thank the following professionals for critiquing sections and chapters of the book, and using their knowledge and experience to ensure that the information included is as accurate as possible.

- Dr Maggie Allen, consultant rheumatologist for the UHCW NHS Trust Coventry, honorary senior lecturer at Warwick Medical School, foundation years generic skills lead for Coventry and Warwickshire Foundation School and chair of the West Midlands Rheumatology Training Committee.
- Mr Mohamed Arafa, consultant orthopaedic surgeon, associate postgraduate dean at West Midlands Deanery and honorary senior clinical lecturer.
- Dr Colin Campbell, consultant paediatrician at the University Hospital of North Staffordshire and associate postgraduate dean of the West Midlands Deanery.
- Mr Paul Deemer, information and intelligence manager for the Equality and Diversity Team, NHS Employers.
- Dr Rose Johnson, consultant in A&E, Worcestershire Royal Hospital.
- Mrs Janet Monkman, chief executive of the South Warwickshire General Hospitals NHS Trust.
- Mr Manjit Obhrai, consultant in obstetrics and gynaecology at the University Hospital of North Staffordshire and postgraduate clinical tutor for the West Midlands Deanery.

Thank you, too, to the following people for their additional input: Dr Helen Goodyear, consultant paediatrician and associate postgraduate dean for flexible training in the West Midlands Deanery; Mrs Clare Kennedy, careers project manager for the West Midlands Deanery; Dr Chris Nancollas, GP; and Helen Westall, final-year medical student at Barts and the London Medical School, and 2005 Trauma Conference organiser.

Most of the illustrations used throughout the book were designed and drawn by Elizabeth Cottrell.

Reference

1   Anderson C and Binding C. *Nottingham Medical School Career Handbook* (2e). Nottingham: Trent Postgraduate Deanery and the University of Nottingham; 2005.

1

Introduction

At graduation, over half of new doctors do not know what specialty they want to enter[1] and many subsequently change career direction. In addition, 55% of doctors report that they are quite or very dissatisfied with the career advice and guidance they have received. Furthermore, 17% say a lack of advice led them to making decisions in their training they now regret.[2] Key messages, discovered following a study of pre-registration house officers' (now known as Foundation Year 1 doctors (F1s)) career intentions, are shown in Box 1.1.[3]

Box 1.1: Key messages arising as a result of a survey of pre-registration house officers (PRHOs)

- Most PRHOs have decided upon their future career within six months of qualification.
- The intention to do general practice falls off during the PRHO year.
- PRHOs prefer to seek advice on the internet and from Sci45, a computer-based career advice tool, than from career advisers.[3]
- The strongest influence on their choice of career was their own experience.
- 'Tasters' and career advice should be offered as early as possible.

This *Handbook* aims to give you, as medical students and junior doctors, the tools you need to start making your own informed career decisions.

As a result of changes in career structures and initiatives such as *Modernising Medical Careers* (MMC) doctors are required to have a pro-active and informed approach to career development. Medical students and doctors have to make career decisions early as specialty training starts just two years after graduation from medical school (after your Foundation training; *see* Chapter 7), therefore you must start thinking about your future medical career while you are still a student. Improving the quality of career information, advice and counselling is vital if the MMC reforms and postgraduate training programmes are to be successful.

No one can make career decisions for you. You have to learn how to help yourself to make informed career choices. This *Handbook* gives you help, tips, advice and signposts for further guidance for embarking on a successful and personally appropriate career.

Why should you read this handbook?

- There is less time to make career decisions than you think.
- It will alert you to the facilities and resources that are available.
- It is a source of reliable and consistent information to help you make an informed decision.

- It gives application advice and help with CVs.
- It contains specialty profiles and job statistics.
- It helps you discover your personality type and therefore which specialty may suit you.
- It informs you of the career advice and support available and how to access these.
- It alerts you to ongoing medical career changes under the MMC initiative.
- It is an interactive resource full of ideas and support for early career development and will be useful right through your junior doctor (Foundation) years – so keep it safe!

Useful texts and websites containing information about career development and useful contact details can be found at the end of each chapter and in Appendix 1. The web addresses provided were correct, and in use, at the time of writing.

Finally, this handbook is accessible through the West Midlands Deanery website (www.wmdeanery.org). You can print the interactive forms in order to complete them.

References

1 Anderson C and Binding C. *Nottingham Medical School Career Handbook* (2e). Nottingham: Trent Postgraduate Deanery and the University of Nottingham; 2005.

2 Jackson C, Ball J and Hirsh W. *Informing Choices: the need for career advice in medical training.* Cambridge: National Institute for Careers Education and Counselling; 2004.

3 Stern C. Career intentions of preregistration house officers and the influence of career advice. *Br J Hosp Med.* 2005; **66**: 477–9.

Further reading

Agha R. *Making Sense of Your Medical Career: your strategic guide to success.* London: Hodder Education; 2005.

Blundell A, Harrison R and Turney B. *The Essential Guide to Becoming a Doctor.* London: BMJ Publishing Group; 2004.

British Medical Association. *Becoming a Doctor: entry in 2005.* London: BMA Board of Medical Education; 2004.

British Medical Association.*BMA Cohort Study of 1995 Medical Graduates. 9th Report.* London: BMA; 2004.

Eccles S and Ward C. *So You Want to Be a Brain Surgeon.* Oxford: Oxford University Press; 2001.

Hopkins D. *So You Want to Be a Doctor: an insider's guide to career opportunities.* London: Kogan Page; 1998.

Hutton-Taylor S. Do it yourself career guidance. *BMJ Careers.* 1996; **313**: 2.

Johnson C, Forrest F and Hall C. *Getting Ahead in Medicine. A Guide to Personal Skills for Doctors.* Oxford: Bios Publishers; 1998.

Royal College of Physicians. *Careers Information Handbook for Trainees.* London: RCP; 2002.

2

Experiences of others

Career pathways are different for everyone. This chapter contains information, lessons and advice from people at various stages of their career.

Below are a few experiences of career development from people at various stages of the medical career pathway. Read and reflect on these experiences and see how you can use them to further your career and make appropriate decisions that suit your circumstances. Compare your own experiences with the ones below. Use the comparison constructively to assess how you have got to where you are and to think about avenues you have not considered previously.

Name: Dr Carol Gray
Position: A&E Consultant; Clinical Dean of Undergraduate Medicine, Keele University
Year of graduation: 1982
University of graduation: University of London (Barts)
Highlights of your career: My present job combination takes a lot of beating, although permanent exhaustion is a drawback!
Problems with career development decisions/bad advice: As a junior doctor I struggled with my primary surgical exams. I went to the surgeon appointed by the college for career advice. After listening to me he suggested I give up and also clearly stated that he felt women who did surgery were frustrated singletons: 'At least you are married' was his comment on seeing my wedding ring. Needless to say, I ignored him and achieved my FRCS (A&E) a couple of years later.
Advice to students about career development: Be realistic. Try to find a career path that really excites you (it helps on bad days) but think about what you want out of the rest of your life as well. If you need time off to study, take it. A short period of locums will not hurt and without exams you will not progress. Be honest at job interviews, it usually pays off. Think about how you will feel when you are finally trained and doing the job day after day – it is very different from being a trainee. Also, develop your non-clinical medical skills. My job is about one-third medical education and the rest as an NHS clinician and I think increasingly this is a model for the future, whether education, research, management or other activities are your 'thing'. A change is frequently as good as a rest!

Name: Dr Sharon Turner
Position: GP
Year of graduation: 1986
University of graduation: Birmingham University
Highlights of your career: Family medicine programme, Illawarra Health Authority, NSW, Australia. Joining current practice; becoming a trainer.
Problems with career development decisions/bad advice: I do not remember getting any bad advice.
Good advice received: Work part-time if you can when children are small and do not take long breaks.
Advice to students about career development: Be open-minded. Try and get a broad experience at junior level. Consider working abroad.

Name: Dr Graham Heyes
Position: Senior House Officer
Year of graduation: 2001
University of graduation: University of Manchester
Highlights of your career: Trauma surgery elective in Montreal General Hospital; A&E six-month Senior House Officer (SHO) post at North Staffordshire General Hospital.
Problems with career development decisions/bad advice: The problem-based learning (PBL) course seems to make it very difficult to pass the MRCP. Hardly anyone in my year has, so far, managed to pass it yet. Going to St Andrews seems to be beneficial to passing the MRCP, a postgraduate exam for those specialising in the medical field. I have had to virtually restart learning medicine (by learning lists as for conventional courses) to enable me to make any headway with passing the exams.
Good advice received: Do some A&E, as it gives you confidence about discharging and admitting patients, although it can be stressful at the time and can impair your social life. Buy a house as soon as you can near a hospital. You can always rent it out later.
Advice to students about career development: Better to delay your choice about SHO rotation (surgery, medicine, anaesthesia) until you are sure rather than getting on a path that you are unsure about.

Name: Dr Fady Magdy
Position: Foundation Year 1 (F1)
Year of graduation: 2005
University of graduation: University of Manchester
Highlights of your career: None stated.
Problems with career development decisions/bad advice: Never had any problems. I knew early on which specialty I wanted to pursue and so I have tailored my undergraduate experience and projects to suit this. I have also chosen suitable rotations for my F1 to gain experience in related specialties.
Good advice received: I received excellent advice from my educational supervisor regarding the experience necessary.
Advice to students about career development: *Be pro-active*. Ask advice from various consultants.

Name: Mr Ravin Ramtohal
Position: Final-year medical student
Year of graduation: (hopefully) 2006
University of graduation: Southampton University Medical School
Highlights of your career: Founding the Southampton medics squash club. I particularly enjoyed the third- and fourth-year attachments, especially dermatology, orthopaedics and ophthalmology.
Problems with career development decisions/ bad advice: Applying for F1 positions was particularly difficult without help from the university.
Good advice received: Third-year pastoral tutor is excellent in her advice in dealing with the pressures of the course.
Advice to students about career development: Build your portfolio and CV, especially aspects that include teamwork and leadership skills.

3

Career development toolkit

This book has been designed to give you the information and skills required to make career decisions and to succeed in the career path you choose. This chapter explicitly provides you with these. The information provided here will assist you in making early career decisions and explain further how to use this book. In addition, with the assistance of information derived from articles produced by Anita Houghton and the Myers–Briggs Type Index (MBTI), this chapter will help you to understand yourself better. Use the information and understanding to pursue an appropriate career.

Advice for managing your career development

You may not have thought much about your career. However, it is never too soon to start doing something about it.

The most important thing you can do is to *be pro-active* – your career will not just happen. To be successful in developing a career plan we advise you to:

- listen to others you are working with
- not be afraid to ask questions, people are generally very happy to talk about their jobs
- take career development opportunities
- seek out help when required
- ask your university if you would like the staff to do, or organise, something for you and your peers; for example, career fairs
- continually appraise your career choices objectively.

An immense amount of information is out there. Information can be gained by reading journals regularly. This will keep you up to date with current practice; journals can often provide career ideas or points for thought. If you have a specific area of interest it is probably worth looking through a few relevant journals before handing over the cash for a subscription. Table 3.1 illustrates the 2006 subscription costs of some of the most popular and useful journals to provide a rough idea of price and affordability.

Table 3.1: Journal subscription costs 2006

Journal	Student subscription	Full-price subscription p.a.	Offers
BMJ International[1]	–	£158	Can receive this in place of the StudentBMJ in final year of study for the StudentBMJ price
StudentBMJ[1]	£35	–	–
BMJ Online[1]	–	–	£23.50 introductory offer
Casebook[2]	Free to MPS* members – membership is free for students	Free to MPS* members – MPS membership is £10 F1 doctor, £40 F2 doctors[3]	Free to MPS* members
Medicine[4]	–	£112	Free for a year then half-price if student
Surgery or Psychiatry[4]	–	£118	Free for a year then half-price if student
Anaesthesia and Intensive Care[4]	–	£124	Free for a year then half-price if student
Women's Health[4]	–	–	£57 new publication offer
The Lancet[5]	–	–	~£20 ($30) for basic package
Clinical Evidence[6]:			
concise and online	£45	£101	
Full edition and online	£51	£111	
Foundation years resource:[7] 12 issues of Medicine and six issues of The Foundation Years journal per year	–	£104	£52 if a MPS* member

* MPS = Medical Protection Society

All university and hospital libraries should have a good selection of medical, medical career or related journals; if not they should be able to obtain any requested. In addition, electronic versions of many journals can be obtained through the National electronic Library for Health (NeLH) (www.nelh.nhs.uk).

The aim of the NeLH is to provide clinicians, medical students, patients, carers and the general public with access to the best current know-how and knowledge to support healthcare-related decisions.

The main priority for the NeLH is to help the National Health Service (NHS) to achieve its objectives. However, it is also useful for healthcare professionals who are working in the private sector where common standards should apply. Part of the content of the NeLH, such as Clinical Evidence and the Cochrane Library, is licensed from commercial providers. Professionals working in public health or social care, or those who are interested in these areas, may find the National Electronic Library for Public Health (www.phel.gov.uk) useful. This website has been developed by the Health Development Agency for all public health professionals, many of whom work in local government. You should make time to investigate these resources as they may not only help with your studies but also with your future career decisions and management.

Getting interactive

Throughout this book you will be told that thinking about your future career cannot start early enough. You should learn to take a critical and reflective look at your motivation, skills and aptitudes to help assist your career progression. Not only that, but career development is an ongoing process which evolves and progresses with each learning experience. To help support your career development, reflection and contemplation, photocopy and complete the forms found in appendices 2 and 3. For the most beneficial results, complete these in your own time and as honestly as possible.

We suggest that the 'Current career interests' form (*see* Appendix 2) is best completed at the following times:

- beginning of third year (first clinical year)
- end of third year (first clinical year)
- end of fourth year (second clinical year)
- end of fifth year (third clinical year)
- end of Foundation Year 1
- end of Foundation Year 2.

We also suggest you complete the 'Using clinical attachments to further career development decisions' form (*see* Appendix 3) after:

- each placement or rotation
- each student-selected component
- your elective.

Each form takes only a few minutes to complete and this will be time well spent. Simply reading the forms and providing answers will stimulate you to consider your current career development situation and assist with job applications in the future.

Specialty profile key

Throughout this *Handbook* you will find profiles of professionals who work in different specialties. Whether or not you have decided what to do with your career, these may provide you with vital information. Each profile contains the following.

This is the current length of the Certificate of Completion of Training (CCT).

Described as low (L), medium (M), high (H) or not available (?), this is the level of competition for each specialty, based on data from *BMJ Careers*[8] and the West Midlands Deanery.[9] For updated information on future levels of competition for different specialties refer to the NHS Professionals website (www.nhsprofessionals.nhs.uk) and the Deanery websites (accessible through www.mmc.nhs.uk).

The amount of out-of-hours work you will be expected to perform as a junior doctor, described as low (+), medium (++), high (+++), fixed shift (F) or variable (V).[9,10]

The following headings will also be found.

- **General overview of specialty**: gives you an idea about the particular specialty.
- **Daily activities**: provides a realistic view of what is involved in the specialty from day to day.
- **Qualities required**: this allows you to match your own qualities, discovered by using the interactive forms, to those required in the specialty. This enables personal assessment of your suitability to the specialty described.
- **Pros and cons**: the good and bad points of the job straight from the doctor's mouth.
- **Sub-specialties**: specialties that fall under the umbrella term of the specialty described.
- **Allied specialties**: specialties that will provide you with similar, related and/or useful additional experience. This can be used for assistance with making choices for student-selected components or electives.
- **Royal College website address**: full details of royal colleges are provided in Appendix 4.

How competitive is your desired specialty?

At present there are over 65 specialties, but how competitive is it out there?

BMJ Careers recently looked at competition rates for junior posts.[8] Pre-registration house officers (PRHOs; now known as Foundation Year 1 doctors, F1), senior house officers (SHOs; now known as Foundation Year 2 doctors, F2), Foundation (F1 and F2) and trust posts across the UK that were advertised in *BMJ Career Focus* from June 2004 to January 2005 were followed up by a questionnaire. These were sent out to the hospitals asking how many vacancies had been advertised and how many applications had been received. Figure 3.1 shows the level of competition as the average number of applications per vacant post.

The study suggests that competition for junior posts is fierce, with A&E posts being the most popular. Competition levels were greatest in Wales and the south-east of England and, surprisingly, lowest in London and Northern Ireland. Competition ratios, specialty descriptions, the attractions, the necessary qualification requirements and the directions to more detailed advice can also be found on both the London and West Midlands Deanery websites (*see* Appendix 1) within the career sections. Do not forget that competition for junior posts may not reflect competition at more senior levels in any specialty. Indeed, competition ratios may be set to change with the reforms in training. There is currently not enough similar data corresponding to F1/F2 competition for each specialty.

A longitudinal survey carried out by junior doctors (PRHOs/F1s and SHOs/F2s) working in Staffordshire looked at junior doctors' preferences for different specialties as career options.[11] Medical specialties were most popular, followed by surgical specialties then anaesthetics, A&E and general practice. The issues that influenced junior doctors' career choice included (in order of preference) anticipated enjoyment, career prospects and working environment.

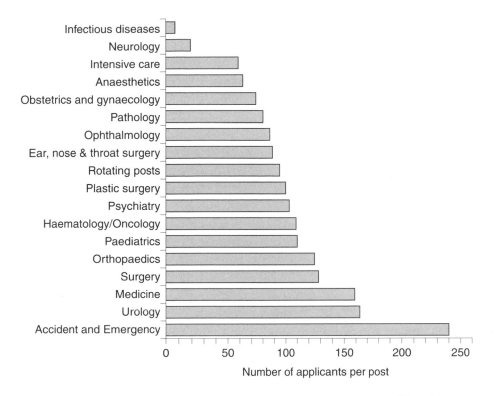

Figure 3.1: Level of competition for junior (PRHO/F1 and SHO/F2) hospital-based posts, 2004/2005.

Specialty profile: Academic medicine

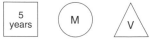

Name: Professor Ruth Chambers

Position: Director of Postgraduate General Practice Education at West Midlands Deanery, Professor of Primary Care at Staffordshire University, GP.

Where have you carried out your research? 1988: Part-time research fellow at Keele University, progressing to be part-time senior lecturer. 1995: Completed my MD (Doctorate) thesis, which I gained from the University of Nottingham. 1997: Professor of Primary Care at Staffordshire University. I have teams of staff to work on research and development projects with me. I work with academics from other institutions across the UK and overseas, and with colleagues from different specialties at my own university. Throughout I have remained as a GP, working full-time until 1997, and since then for one or two sessions per week.

Daily activities: Attracting research funding; agreeing the research and development protocol; applying for ethics and research governance approval;

---

appointing the team and generally overseeing that we are fulfilling the research protocol; writing up research for a peer-reviewed journal.

Qualities required: Self-belief in your ability is vital; a wide base of knowledge and skills; the ability to teach; good communication skills.

Opportunities: You can make academic medicine your main career or a fringe activity, work with the Royal College of your specialty, travel the world, use your research or teaching materials to write books. I have done all of these and am now on my 58th book.

Advice to interested students: Gain experience by helping the research department in your teaching hospital gather data as part of an ongoing research study.

Competition for posts in different specialties will change in the future as the new *Modernising Medical Careers* initiative is established (*see* Chapter 7). In addition, competition for different specialties varies according to year of training and year by year. The ratios of applicants to available posts are usually completely different for doctors entering specialty or GP training to the competition for PRHO/F1 and SHO/F2 posts. Therefore, you must investigate the most recently published competition information for different specialties for the level of training that applies to you. Updated information on levels of competition for different specialties may be found on the NHS Professionals website (www.nhsprofessionals.nhs.uk) and the postgraduate deanery websites (accessible through www.mmc.nhs.uk).

Matching personality type to career

Analysing your personality may fill you with fear. You may be worried you will discover a hidden secret! Maybe you feel uncomfortable with the potential for being labelled or stereotyped, or both? However, understanding your personality can benefit both you as a medic and your patients. This will be explained, using work by Anita Houghton and information based on the Myers–Briggs Type Indicator (MBTI). Houghton states that by understanding and evaluating your personal style and preferences you will quickly and more easily be able to understand and better value others. As a result you will have increased productivity, improved working relationships and a happier, more fulfilled working life.[12] The main themes of the MBTI are described in more detail below.

Whatever your opinion of psychometric testing, start getting used to such assessments. From 2006, students wanting to study medicine at the universities of Glasgow, Edinburgh, Aberdeen, St Andrew's and Dundee will sit personality and mental agility tests; these aim to identify which candidates are best suited to a career in medicine.[13] As the BMA medical students' committee is broadly supportive of psychometric testing as part of the application process, it may soon spread to other universities as part of their medical school admissions procedure.

The Open University has produced an interactive CD-ROM package that uses another form of psychometric testing. The *Sci45*, specialty choice inventory, requires the user to comment on 130 statements designed to identify which of 80 job attributes are valued most highly. This is then correlated to job suitability, helping you to select a specialty that best fits with your own attitudes, aspirations, academic orientation and personal characteristics.[14]

The MBTI is a framework that describes four areas in which people differ (extroversion/introversion, sensing/intuition, thinking/feeling and judging/perceiving) and labels personality depending on these differences. The MBTI is a well-endorsed and frequently used psychometric test, hence it deserves further explanation.[15]

Your 'type' is merely a collection of approaches or practices that you prefer to carry out, which only you can identify. In reality, these preferred approaches co-exist so we express more than one personality type in different settings and circumstances. However, we usually display a single dominating preference for a particular 'type'. These preferred approaches are nothing to do with our abilities, which are a completely separate issue. It is important to realise that we can all be taught approaches or practices preferred by our opposing types.

Specialty profile: Accident and emergency

| 5 years | (M–H) | /F\ |

Name: Dr Arvinder Sadana
Position: Consultant in Emergency Medicine (A&E)
Hospital: St George's, London
Daily activities: Vary enormously, but supervision of junior staff is the most important and enjoyable part. Teaching, administration and meetings comprise most of the time. Typically, I start work between 8 am and 8.30 am, attend an escalation meeting for 10–15 minutes, assess the 'state' of the department, perform 'shop floor' work or do administration or teaching, etc. I usually leave at around 6 pm.
Qualities required: Ability to 'multi-task', flexibility/adaptability, sense of humour, ability to stay calm at all (well, most) times.
Pros: Interesting, challenging and unpredictable work; a lot of flexibility; good team spirit.
Cons: These change, but currently pressures imposed by central government to meet targets seem to override other priorities.
Sub-specialties: Recognised sub-specialties in the UK are paediatrics and intensive care. Most A&E consultants will have their own particular interests; mine are toxicology, acute medicine and observation wards.
Allied specialties: Most other specialties are useful but, in particular, general medicine, cardiology, anaesthetics/ITU, paediatrics, orthopaedics and some general surgery.
Royal College website address: www.rcplondon.ac.uk

So, what is your type? Read the statements in Table 3.2, 'Personality toolkit', and tick only those that you honestly believe describe you. Then refer to Figure 3.2 and follow the flowchart based on the answers you ticked to find out what personality type you predominantly are. Figure 3.2 also highlights some of the traits that constitute that type: qualities that you may discover describe you accurately. Reflect on these traits; can you identify them within yourself? Had you realised you owned these traits before?

Table 3.2: Personality toolkit

1a	I really enjoy teamwork and mixing with lots of people at work/ university/socially	
1b	I like days when I have the chance to read, reflect, study or write	
1c	If a new person joins the firm/group I'm the first one to approach them, welcome them and invite them to tonight's social event	
1d	On a ward round, when the firm is asked a question, I think through my answer carefully before speaking	
1e	A day full of action and interacting with loads of people is draining	
2a	I prefer lectures/talks to provide information in a detailed, stepwise and factual manner	
2b	I am always full of new ideas, different ways of doing things and focus on tomorrow	
2c	When given data I like to create patterns and meanings associated with it, and develop theories and possibilities	
2d	I trust experience and tried and tested methods of doing things	
2e	If someone were to ask me to describe an object I would give a precise description of what it looks like and its exact function	
3a	I make decisions based on what is the most logical thing to do rather than how it will affect others involved	
3b	People describe me as reasonable, fair and objective, and I like to be complimented for my competency	
3c	I enjoy talking to patients and relatives	
3d	People describe me as compassionate, tender and kind, and I like to be complimented for these qualities	
3e	I am guided by values rather than cause and effect	
4a	I like to have a clear plan of what I am doing and when, to have organisation and structure in my life	
4b	I adapt to change easily, I am good in emergencies and filling in at the last minute	
4c	I like being prepared and getting jobs done	
4d	I feel constrained by schedules and like to keep my options open	
4e	I am flexible, spontaneous, and feel energised by last-minute pressures	

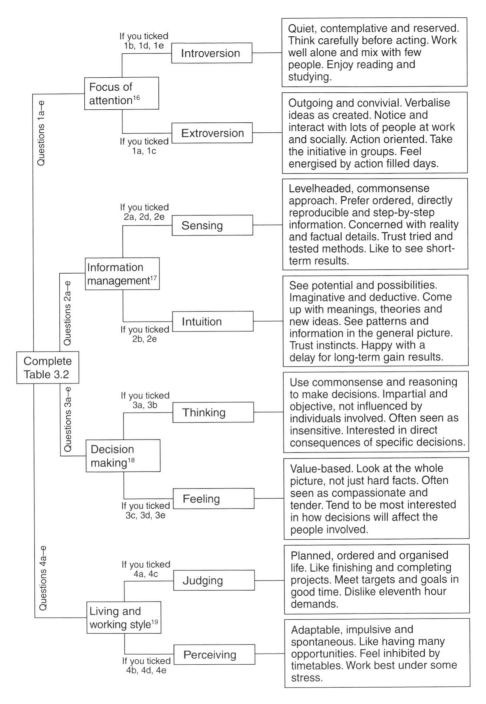

Figure 3.2:   Working out your predominant personality type.

Once you have discovered your predominant personality type you can use this information constructively to assist you in maximising your efficiency and efficacy at work. Houghton identified a number of tasks and activities that take place every day in medicine, which are presented in Figure 3.3. Knowing which of these are preferred by your personality type allows you to consider the areas of medicine in which your strengths lie and, therefore, which future career may best suit you.

Advice for dealing with activities requiring non-predominant personality traits

The range of activities carried out by each personality type, shown in Figure 3.3, illustrates the point that you cannot practise medicine without using opposing approaches on a daily basis. For example, we all have to learn to take systematic clinical histories (preferred by sensing types) whilst at medical school yet we need intuition to look at all the information the patient gives us, to think of possible differential diagnoses, create hypotheses and make a final diagnosis. Being predominantly one type rather than the other just means that some activities will be easier. Engaging in these preferred activities will be exciting and you will be enthusiastic about them, whereas engaging in non-preferred activities will tend to exhaust and consume you. It is often difficult to understand opposite preference types, especially when they seem so different to your own. In addition, you may feel hindered or unappreciated in a job where you have to spend a considerable amount of time carrying out activities preferred by your opposing personality type. So how do you cope with such activities? Read on!

You may now have more idea of what your main preferences are, and what activities you are likely to prefer carrying out. So how do you cope with the tasks you are not so good at, or dislike doing?

- Value people with other personality types:
  - understand and respect that everyone is different
  - recognise that each type has qualities and strengths
  - try and get help from a person of a different personality type to maximise your efficiency
  - if you are having trouble acting outside your type ask the opposing type how they would deal with the same situation.
- Do activities preferred by your non-predominant, opposing type when you are best able to cope with them:
  - understand what times of day and in which situations you are at your most alert and when you are at your weakest
  - arrange to undertake non-preferred activities, as described in Figure 3.3, when you are at your strongest
  - do non-preferred activities frequently but in small bursts so they do not build up.
- Tailor your job applications to your own personal preferences:
  - identify aspects of your current work or rotations you do not enjoy and decide if your personality type can explain why
  - obtain a copy of the job description and make a note of activities that you are really good at and enjoy

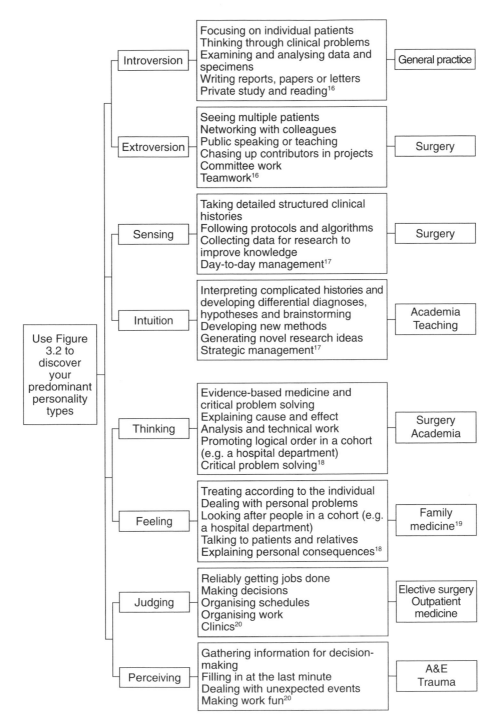

Figure 3.3: Examples of components and areas of medicine suited to particular personality types.

- think carefully about any jobs you are applying for and how much of your non-preferred activities they will involve; those containing more of your preferred activities will make you happier and more fulfilled
- remember your type when applying for jobs; use your known strengths and qualities to promote yourself on your application forms
- think carefully about any specialties you would like to work in and the activities these include.
- Redress the balance after a day engaged in your non-preferred activities:
  - do activities that best suit your predominant personality types – *see* figures 3.2 and 3.3 for ideas!

You will now have a good idea of your personality preferences. Although these personal preferences are described separately, in reality they co-exist and it is the hugely variable interaction between each of them that determines your overall personality type. According to MBTI there are 16 personality types formed from combinations of the different indices (for example, ISTJ, ESTP, INFJ) influencing your reactions to different situations.[21]

If this section has interested you in discovering more about your personality type, all 16 type descriptions may be found on a website (www.capt.org/mbti-assessment/type-descriptions.htm) and further references can be found in Appendix 1.

What is the best personality type to be? For you, the type you really are. The most rewarding experiences you have will be those that come through the strengths that constitute your personality type.[22] Just remember that preferred approaches to thinking, acting and decision-making are not abilities. We can all be taught approaches or practices that are outside those we prefer when the situation demands.

Intelligent career card sort

A career exploration tool is being piloted in the Trent Multi-Professional Deanery. Individuals select statements on cards that make up the Intelligent Career Card Sort (ICCS).[23] They choose the ones that best reflect how they think of their current career situation. The three different-coloured cards are divided into three ways of 'knowing':

- Knowing *why* (blue): about knowing yourself, your motivations and values, and how you relate to your career.
- Knowing *how* (yellow): knowing about the skills you possess or those you want to develop.
- Knowing *whom* (green): allows you to reflect on the relationships and reputations you have, or the connections you would like to make.

All three categories link closely together, as seen in Figure 3.4, and form the basis of a series of consultations facilitated by someone trained in the use and application of the framework (an ICCS consultant). The technique requires several hours' attention and work over a period of time.

The system is based on the idea that individuals are in charge of their own career progression. Individuals should reflect on a range of different options available. No definitive advice is given, nor is a particular career choice suggested. It is more about providing you with an opportunity to learn about yourself and how this will direct your future career endeavours. If you would like to find out more about this career tool you can visit the website (www.intelligentcareer.com) or contact the guidance and support associate at Trent Multi-Professional Deanery.

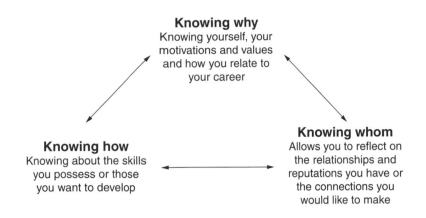

Figure 3.4:   Ways in which the 'knowing' categories are related.

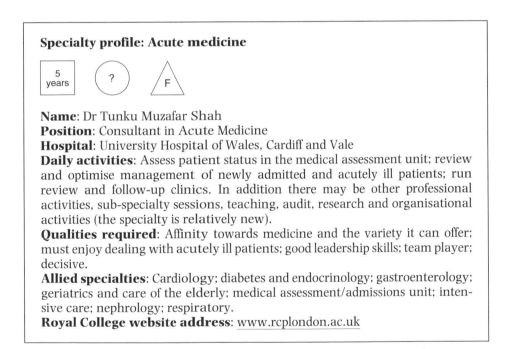

Specialty profile: Acute medicine

Name: Dr Tunku Muzafar Shah
Position: Consultant in Acute Medicine
Hospital: University Hospital of Wales, Cardiff and Vale
Daily activities: Assess patient status in the medical assessment unit; review and optimise management of newly admitted and acutely ill patients; run review and follow-up clinics. In addition there may be other professional activities, sub-specialty sessions, teaching, audit, research and organisational activities (the specialty is relatively new).
Qualities required: Affinity towards medicine and the variety it can offer; must enjoy dealing with acutely ill patients; good leadership skills; team player; decisive.
Allied specialties: Cardiology; diabetes and endocrinology; gastroenterology; geriatrics and care of the elderly; medical assessment/admissions unit; intensive care; nephrology; respiratory.
Royal College website address: www.rcplondon.ac.uk

References

1   www.bmjjournals.com/subscriptions/

2   www.medicalprotection.org/medical/united_kingdom/publications/casebook/

3   www.medicalprotection.org/medical/united_kingdom/membership/
    subscription_rates/hospital_2005.aspx

4   www.medicinejournal.co.uk

5   www.lancet.com

6   www.bmjjournals.com/subscriptions/cepers2006.pdf

7   www.medicinepublishing.co.uk/index.php/foundationyears

8   www.bmjcareers.com

9   www.wmdeanery.org/careerguide/foreword.htm

10 Eccles S and Ward C. *So You Want to Be a Brain Surgeon* (2e). Oxford: Oxford University
    Press; 2001.

11 Davidson I, Bullock A and Burke S. *A Supplement to the Final Report: careers advice for junior
    doctors: a longitudinal survey from the second year of the Staffordshire Pilot Careers Advice
    Service*. Birmingham: School of Education, University of Birmingham; 2005.

12 Houghton A. Understanding personality type: introduction. *StudentBMJ*. 2004; **12**: 366–7.

13 StudentBMA. MSC ticks 'unsure' for personality testing plan. *StudentBMA News*. 2005;
    Dec: 2.

14 Gale R and Grant J. *Sci45 Specialty Choice Inventory: computer-based careers advice for
    doctors in training*. Milton Keynes: Open University Centre for Education in Medicine;
    2002.

15 Bess TL and Harvey RJ. Bimodal score distributions and the Myers–Briggs type indicator:
    fact or artefact. *J Pers Asses*. 2002; **78**: 176–86.

16 Houghton A. Understanding personality type: extraversion and introversion. *StudentBMJ*.
    2004; **12**: 410–11.

17 Houghton A. Understanding personality type: sensing and intuition. *StudentBMJ*. 2004;
    12: 456–7.

18 Houghton A. Understanding personality type: how do you make decisions. *StudentBMJ*.
    2005; **13**: 20–1.

19 Stilwell NA, Wallick MM, Thal SE et al. Myers–Briggs type and medical specialty choice:
    a new look at an old question. *Teach Learn Med*. 2000; **12**: 14–20.

20 Houghton A. Understanding personality type: how do you like to live your life.
    StudentBMJ. 2005; **13**: 62–3.

21 Houghton A. Understanding personality type: how it relates to job satisfaction.
    StudentBMJ. 2005; **13**: 108–9.

22 www.capt.org/mbti-assessment/best-type.htm

23 Binding C and Loveland M. Career choice: your future on the cards. *BMJ Careers*. 2005;
    331: 197–9.

Further reading

Chambers R, Mohanna K and Field S. *Opportunities and Options in Medical Careers*. Oxford: Radcliffe Medical Press; 2000.

Hopson B and Scally M. *Build Your Own Rainbow: workbook for career and life management* (2e). London: Kogan Page; 2000.

Houghton A. *Know Yourself: the individual's guide to career development in healthcare*. Oxford: Radcliffe Publishing; 2005.

Kendell E. *The Myers–Briggs Type Indicator Manual: UK supplement*. Oxford: Oxford Psychologists Press; 1998.

MacKinnon DW. Personality and the realization of creative potential. *Am Psych*. 1965; **20**: 273–81.

Myers IB and McCaulley MH. *MBTI Manual: a guide to the development and use of the Myers–Briggs type indicator* (3e). Palo Alto, CA: Consulting Psychologists Press; 1998.

Research centre for the Myers–Briggs type index (www.capt.org).

4

Career support, advisers and fairs

There are many opportunities available for you to obtain help and further information on career decisions and options. This chapter is designed to highlight the resources available to you.

Career support

Access to career advice for both undergraduate students and postgraduate doctors has been limited in the past. Historically, the lack of appropriate career guidance has been well documented.[1] Most doctors report that they have never received any career guidance or counselling.[2] In a survey of British Medical Association (BMA) members, consisting of doctors and medical students, 95% of respondents reported that they had unmet career guidance requirements.[3]

Specialty profile: Age-related medicine

3 years	L	+- ++

Name: Dr A Y Chaudhry
Position: Consultant Physician in Acute Medicine and Gerontology Department
Hospital: Walsgrave Hospital UHCW NHS Trust, Coventry
Daily activities: Ward round for inpatients three times per week, outpatients clinics and multi-disciplinary team meetings, teaching, academic meetings and meeting with relatives.
Qualities required: Good time management skills are essential. An understanding of what the job entails, as it can be frustrating when you are very busy and your contemporaries are having time free. Good communication skills, particularly with relatives.
Pros: Excellent opportunity to learn acute medicine along with basic practical procedures; good team spirit; opportunities for involvement in audit and academic activities; excellent opportunity for holistic approach to patient care.

Cons: Very busy job; frustrating delayed discharges due to community social issues.

Sub-specialties: Falls; transient ischaemic attacks (TIAs); stroke; rehabilitation; Parkinson's disease.

Allied specialties: Orthogeriatric; geriatric psychiatry; palliative care.

Students would be advised to consider part-time work (e.g. as a healthcare assistant) in this specialty if you have not had previous exposure.

Royal College website address: www.rcplondon.ac.uk; British Geriatric Society (www.bgs.org.uk).

The document *Signposting Medical Careers for Doctors*[4] highlights the recent situation; few medical students and doctors have access to impartial career advice and counselling, and they make career decisions based on 'preconceptions rather than sound judgement'.[4] They are often not aware what is actually available or where to go for advice. Traditionally, career advice has been sought in an informal, ad hoc manner. In a survey of BMA members that included an assessment of views on previous career advice, respondents reported their views as indicated in Table 4.1.

Table 4.1: Results from the survey of BMA members on the helpfulness of career advice[3]

Source of advice	Ratings	Percentage
More experienced peers	Useful or very useful	93
Senior doctors	Useful or very useful	87
Doctors who are family or friends	Useful or very useful	83
Peer group members	Useful or very useful	80
BMJ Career Focus	Useful or very useful	79
University career advice	Useful	41
Medical career fairs	Useful	44
Career lectures at medical school	Useful	40

Both students and institutions should adopt a pro-active and educational approach to career advice and guidance,[3] which should be incorporated into the medical school and Foundation-training curricula. This means that fundamental changes have been, and should continue to be, made to career advice and guidance to make sure it is consistent, structured and clear as to who provides what. Some useful career advice is illustrated in Figure 4.1.

As a result of the recent *Modernising Medical Careers* (MMC) initiative, there has been a great move towards improving the level and standard of career advice made available to medical students and doctors at all levels of training. The provision of career advice is an integral part of the new medical career structure and, hence, thankfully, career support continues to be important as an expanding issue. Changes recently occurring as a result of this include the allocation of funding for a career adviser in each deanery.

Career Management: An Approach for Medical Schools, Deaneries, Royal Colleges and Trusts,[5] produced by the MMC Working Group for Career Management, highlights and suggests potential approaches to the delivery of career management initiatives for doctors between August 2005 and the end of 2007.[6] MMC guidelines (June 2005)[5]

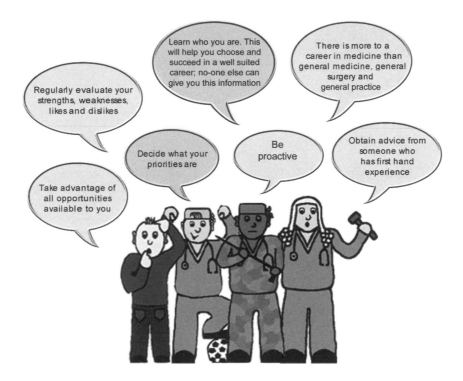

Figure 4.1:   Useful career advice and opportunities.

state that medical schools should be responsible for the delivery of career guidance by providing information and support to students in the following key areas:

- Implementing career management initiatives by integrating them into the medical school curriculum (*see* Chapter 5).
- Developing the knowledge and skills required during undergraduate and postgraduate training.
- Developing the skills required by those giving, or likely to give, career information, advice or guidance.
- Encouraging students and developing their awareness and insight of personal strengths and weaknesses (*see* the 'Current career interests' form in Appendix 2 and the 'Using clinical attachments to further career development decisions' form in Appendix 3) and how these correspond to the variety of career opportunities there are in medicine.

With regard to postgraduate deaneries: these have a responsibility, along with medical schools, to provide support for medical graduates' transition into employment in their two-year Foundation course. You should expect:[6]

- Focused postgraduate curricula activities, including those that broaden your understanding of postgraduate medical education and what it means in practical terms for you.

- Active facilitation and support of career management, with an impartial perspective and advice to signpost and support career networks (online, peer group, one-to-one career activities) which can help progress the continuing career interests and professional aspirations of doctors.
- Access to relevant and accurate sources of information when making a choice of medical career.

Specialty profile: Anaesthetics

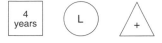

Name: Dr Keith Clayton
Position: Consultant Anaesthetist, Honorary Senior Lecturer University of Warwick; Chair, Hospital Transfusion Committee
Hospital: Walsgrave Hospital and Coventry & Warwick Hospital (C & W)
Daily activities: I usually arrive at C&W at about 7.50 am to see patients and set up for an early start. I aim to finish at about 5 pm with no lunch break. In an average week I will also lecture at the medical school. Throughout the week I work in theatre on a variety of cases, including ophthalmology, breast surgery and orthopaedics. I also work with patients requiring pain relief.
Qualities required: Knowledgeable; team player; good communicator; dextrous; extrovert. Leadership qualities develop over the years.
Pros: Our on-call commitment on the general rota is about one in 20, which is extremely civilised. You pick on-call days which are convenient to you, for example four Mondays and a weekend. You get to work in teams that develop over the years. You can change your sessions over the years – I did 10 years of obstetric anaesthesia before changing my sessions around. It gives you the ability to have a new job every few years. There are opportunities to work in ITU, chronic pain, acute pain, neuro, cardiac, paediatrics – the choices are endless. The opportunity to teach and develop other skills is always encouraged within the department.
Cons: None that I can think of, as long as you like a challenge and are not afraid of hard work.
Sub-specialties: Intensive care: for those who like acute medicine. Chronic pain: for those who like outpatients, with a hint of psychology and practical procedures. Trauma: for those who like to pretend they are in ER. Cardiac, neuro, upper and lower GIT surgery and vascular anaesthesia: for those who like sick patients needing invasive monitoring and excellent pain relief. Day case surgery: for those who like fit patients. Orthopaedics and urology: for those who like elderly patients. Then there are management, teaching, risk management, audit and legal/ethical issues.
Allied specialties: Prior to entry to anaesthesia it is positive to do one year in medicine, paediatrics/neonates, ITU or A&E (or combinations). Once into training you will rotate through all the sub-specialties and then develop your chosen sub-specialty in the last two years of training. Whenever you are doing a surgical attachment come into the anaesthetic room and follow the patient through the complete episode – anaesthetic room, theatre and recovery. Your

insight into patient care will improve. In terms of electives and work experience just enjoy yourself and see life because it is the ability to talk to patients, inform and reassure them, that is essential. Work with the elderly – appreciate their problems and fears. If you are set on a career in anaesthetics do not bother with an F2 job – go for a complementary specialty.
Royal College website address: www.rcoa.ac.uk

These processes are not mutually exclusive. In fact, they form part of the career development continuum. The division of responsibility at different phases in training means that career progression is not always addressed adequately.[3] Good communication, a good framework and commitment to career support is needed by both undergraduate courses and postgraduate deaneries to provide integrated services and prevent fragmentation of advice and guidance. At present there is more of a support structure for Foundation doctors rather than undergraduate medical students, but plans are in place to rectify this situation.

What you should expect

According to *Career Management: An Approach for Medical Schools, Deaneries, Royal Colleges and Trusts*, produced by the MMC Working Group for Career Management,[5] there is a delivery model consisting of 14 components that should provide individuals with all the information, support and confidence needed to make informed and successful career choices. These include the following.

- Career information sources: these should cover job availability and training requirements and qualifications needed for different specialties, competition ratios and personal perspectives of posts (*see* boxed specialty profiles) as well as career pathways.
- Career conferences: events designed for undergraduate medical students and Foundation doctors to learn about different specialties, be involved in workshops (CV, interview, management skills) and debates.
- Career forums: provided as a rolling programme of events covering the main specialties. A career forum is a source of career information and a resource which encourages exploration of career options for senior undergraduates and Foundation doctors.
- Career handbooks: these should cover all the aspects of a career in medicine that are found in this one!
- Online guidance and career discussions: a range of adequately prepared individuals can be contacted to provide information and discuss career topics of interest nationally.
- Peer group activities: for both medical students and Foundation trainees. These provide a supportive career management environment where career exploration, development of skills and, later, discussions on career decisions can take place.
- Specialist career planning tools or programmes: help to develop good career decisions through the use of tools such as the personality toolkit, the 'Current career interests' form, the 'Using clinical attachments to further career development decisions' form and the Sci45.
- Focused experiences: *see* Chapter 6.
- Designated career advisers: *see below*.

- Designated trained career contacts: more targeted one-to-one advice in the form of clinical staff and non-medical professionals – *see below*.
- Medical school support services: integration of career management will be facilitated by student support and guidance through undergraduate, BMA, educational and academic committees and groups, as well as through occupational health, faculty and other pastoral support and guidance.
- Postgraduate deanery guidance and support services: support should be provided for trainees in difficulty through the use of career counselling, career tools and career development advice and facilitating access to a coach or mentor (*see* Chapter 5) and to occupational health or a psychologist when needed.
- Occupational health and occupational psychology: these are a source of external professional advice, especially when a doctor is unable to pursue a specific career option.

Via the MMC initiative, a mechanism is in place to co-ordinate career advice efforts on a national level. The aim is to abolish the current situation, in which there is a huge variety in the services provided by different deaneries. It is hoped, as a result, that experiences will be shared and development costs reduced.

There are a large number of individuals who can provide career advice, information and guidance to medical professionals. Commonly, such individuals are clinical tutors of particular specialties. Key career support organisations also have at least a minimum level of career guidance skills and are aware of best practice in the giving of career information and advice. These are noted in *Career Management: An Approach for Medical Schools, Deaneries, Royal Colleges and Trusts*[5] and include the following.

- Your postgraduate deanery (*see* the MMC website in Appendix 1), including your F1 or F2 programme director, dean and associate dean: these may provide career information, career conferences, a career handbook, online guidance, peer group activities, specialist career planning tools or programmes, focused experiences, career advisers and designated trained career contacts, postgraduate deanery guidance and support services, occupational health and occupational psychology.
- Your medical school deanery, including any university career service that may be in place: these are able to co-ordinate career information, career forums, career conference, career handbook, peer group activities, specialist career planning tools or programmes, focused experiences, career advisers and designated trained career contacts and medical school support services.
- Medical royal colleges (*see* Appendix 4), faculties and institutions.
- Individuals, such as clinical tutors, educational supervisors (*see* Chapter 5), mentors (*see* Chapter 5) and career advisers.
- Career fairs.
- Student-selected components, electives, 'tasters', intercalated degrees, summer jobs, part-time work, work experience (*see* Chapter 6).
- NHS Careers: a good career information source which operates through a national call centre, website and free literature.[7]
- *BMJ Careers*.
- Medical Forum: an independent web service offering help with career planning, management courses, reviews and counselling.[8]
- The Association for Graduate Careers Advisory Services (AGCAS).
- The Institute for Career Guidance (ICG).
- The NHS trust employing you: should provide career information, occupational health and occupational psychology when it is appropriate.

Although the above list is a good starting point, to identify the appropriate organisations or individuals to assist you with career decisions, you should also look on notice
boards, websites and in locally produced booklets for information on where further
career advice can be sought.

Specialty profile: Cardiology

| 6 years | M | △ +++ |

Name: Dr M F Shiu
Position: Consultant Cardiologist
Hospital: University hospitals, Coventry and Warwickshire, Coventry
Daily activities: Average working day is nine hours (excluding travelling). A
typical consultant's week consists of: two outpatient clinics, three to five cardiac
catheter lab sessions, two ward rounds and a half-day for multi-disciplinary
team work. Some ward rounds and clinics have teaching incorporated into
them. Remaining time is used for administration, which includes answering
patient queries, by phone or letter and dictating letters and discharge sum-
maries.
Qualities required: Cardiology has a number of sub-specialties, suiting many
temperaments and skills. Those good with their hands will be suited to coronary
interventions. Conversely, you can specialise in imaging and therapeutics or
hypertension if you like the traditions of a physician.
Pros: Job satisfaction is high; mixture of one-to-one patient care and the use of
new technology for high-tech imaging and treatment; balance between the
one-to-one outpatient work and the group interaction at ward rounds; good
mixture of calm elective work and frantic emergencies.
Cons: Long days; the feeling that the rest of the NHS system is not really up to
date despite efforts at keeping up with the cutting edge of medicine.
Sub-specialties: Interventional (coronary and other cardiac interventions);
imaging (often combined with heart failure); cardiac arrhythmias; cardio-
vascular medicine (often combined with a general medicine accreditation);
grown-up congenital heart disease (a small but important area); academic
cardiology (overlaps clinical and basic science).
Allied specialties: A solid general training in acute general medicine is
essential. Specialties such a nephrology and ITU give excellent experience
with the acutely sick often with multi-system involvement. Overseas electives in
Asia, North America and some parts of Africa would provide a good insight into
the increasingly global nature of the burden of heart disease and give good
preparation for subsequent training.
Royal College website address: www.rcplondon.ac.uk; British Cardiac Society (www.bcs.com).

Career advisers

Funding has recently been given to deaneries to improve career management. One way in which they may do this is to appoint specific career advisers. Many advisers are thus very new to their roles and will be finding their feet, others are still to join and some may already be part of an established system.

According to *Career Management: An Approach for Medical Schools, Deaneries, Royal Colleges and Trusts,*[5] the idea behind the career adviser's role is to:

- provide generic career advice to individual doctors
- respond to the initial career needs of medical undergraduates
- act as a signposting forum and referral point for more complex career-related requirements, such as human resources support
- address situations where no current career advice is being provided
- assist in career exploration through accurate information provision, encouraging reflective career progression and workforce profiling
- use career education and planning tools effectively
- promote consistent practice in screening individuals' readiness to make career decisions.

Career advisers are a useful source of advice and information as they are competent in a range of career management techniques and are aware of accepted good practice.

Designated trained career contacts provide more targeted one-to-one advice. They can give more skilled advice in placement issues, answer specific career queries such as specialty advice and provide targeted training co-ordination for those experiencing particular difficulties. They may also be able to provide confidential in-depth career counselling. In addition, some advisers may be trained in psychometric testing.

The MMC documentation[5] suggests that those who can deliver this service include the following.

- Appropriately qualified clinicians: these may include mentors, educational and clinical supervisors (*see* Chapter 5), clinical tutors, Royal College tutors and advisers, and associate postgraduate deans with specialty career interests.
- Clinical staff: nursing and allied health professionals who have worked closely with medical students and doctors.
- Non-medical professionals: qualified career advisers, experienced facilitators, HR representatives, postgraduate education centre managers and clinical education staff.

The amount of training designated career contacts receive depends on the institute. For example, trainee advisers at the University of Oxford attend a half-day course, whereas the University of Nottingham runs a series of courses covering counselling, career advice, how to access counselling and guidance facilities and stress management. The West Midlands Deanery provides formal training in advice and guidance for all associate deans and is interested in defining competencies for those giving career support.[3]

If you have not yet narrowed down your career choices, you may need to consult several advisers, or an adviser with a broader knowledge of a range of specialties.

Previously there were serious concerns about the advice given by career advisers. These concerns are easy to understand as there was no regular monitoring of the quality of the advice given, nor any effective channel for trainees to voice their concerns.[9] With an explicit framework now in place and at least minimal training for anyone supplying simple factual career advice, as well as more thorough training for those providing in-depth career planning and counselling services, the situation should improve. It must be remembered, however, that not all consultants you discuss career matters with, especially if in an ad hoc fashion, are skilled in appraisal or career counselling[10] and they may provide a biased view and judgemental opinion.[11]

You must learn to evaluate the information anyone gives you. It is also worth noting here that, in a study of the career intentions of pre-registration house officers (PRHOs; now known as Foundation Year 1, F1), web-based career advice and using Sci45 (*see* Chapter 3) were more valued than career advice sessions. In fact, from 89 PRHOs who met either their clinical tutor or another career adviser, 83% found this source of career information or advice the least useful.[12] It is hoped that this view will change with the new reforms.

Career fairs and forums

Local

The newly appointed education supervisors or career advisers should be advertising career fairs, forums and lectures at your university. Through researching local career events it has become obvious, that, as at spring 2006, some of you do not have these. If this is the case – *demand* it! You should never be worried about asking your medical school for help with your career development. Make sure it is providing you with adequate career support, as detailed in the previous section.

Career fairs are not exclusively organised by your medical school directly, but often by medical student societies. For example, surgical societies (known in some medical schools as 'SCRUBS' or 'SCALPEL') may organise career fairs. However, you must either ensure that they are not biased or, if you think they are, take any directed information with a pinch of salt.

Trent Deanery offers an excellent example of how the system should exist. This deanery has held planned optional events for the last seven years following a rolling programme. Supported by the Medical Protection Society (MPS) and the Medical Defence Union (MDU), lectures are run in the evenings in the medical school lecture theatre. These lectures cover a variety of specialties, including medicine, surgery, obstetrics, gynaecology, paediatrics, A&E, anaesthetics and GP career options. Both students and Foundation doctors further benefit from these evenings by having the opportunity to obtain answers to more specific questions and to network with colleagues.

In addition to attending such events you should ensure that advice on CV writing and interview skills are provided too.

Specialty profile: Ear, nose and throat (ENT) surgery

| 6 years | H | ++ |

Name: Mr Paul Wilson
Position: Consultant ENT surgeon
Hospital: University Hospital of North Staffordshire, Stoke-on-Trent
Daily activities: I am not typical of an ENT surgeon! I undertake a mix of clinics and/or operating sessions with some administration during lunch or prior to the start of the day. Clinics may be adult or children, and specialty or general.
Qualities required: As with most clinical posts, good communication skills, empathy, good organisation and time management, dexterity.
Pros: On-call generally relaxed, phone queries mainly, family friendly, OK private practice (at present).
Cons: Busy during daytimes and waiting list pressures.
Sub-specialties: Otology, head and neck cancer, thyroid/parathyroid, laryngology and voice, base of skull.
Allied specialties: Plastic surgery, neurosurgery. Begin by asking juniors doing ENT what they think; undertake an elective in ENT; peer work experience at Foundation level as day release.
Royal College website address: www.rcseng.ac.uk

Regional

PasTest runs a north-west medical recruitment fair. This is the region's only major exhibition for medical career recruitment and education. The event provides the opportunity to meet and discuss career options with over 50 different organisations. It is held at the G-MEX Centre in Manchester in either October or November each year and it is free.[13]

BMJ Careers is also working on a programme to provide regional career fairs next year so keep looking at the website for details.[14]

A multi-deanery career fair was held in the West Midlands in June 2006, for the three West Midlands universities and junior doctors. Look at the MMC website to find out whether there is something similar being held when you need it.

National

Every year the *British Medical Journal* (BMJ) holds a national career fair at the end of November or beginning of December at the Business Design Centre, Islington, London. This is the largest medical recruitment fair in the UK. It runs seminars, provides career advice, helps job seekers and demonstrates new career pathways. You can visit more than 80 exhibition stands representing education, medical recruitment, training, development and advisory organisations. The fair is free to British Medical Association (BMA) members, who can register online (*see* Appendix 1).

Note, there is a charge for the skills builder courses at the fair. These allow you to participate in activities focusing on CV writing and interview skills, time management and decision-making, how to work in teams, how to get what you want and educates you on how to use information technology (IT). In 2005 the charge was £20, but this may increase so you must look it up if you are interested. You can even have a one-to-one session with their carefully selected career advisers for a small fee. Again, in 2005 this fee was £25, but you would have to find out about the cost of this when you attend. All prices and details are on the BMA website.

At the time of printing, annual, summer *BMJ Careers* fairs were being organised for Glasgow (Scotland), Belfast (Northern Ireland) and Cardiff (Wales). These career fairs are similar to the national career fair in Islington. For further details of the year you wish to attend, the full line up of lectures, stalls and prices of skill builder courses, please check information on the website www.bmjcareersfair.com.

The Royal Society of Medicine runs an annual large career and specialty fair in London. The event showcases career options to young doctors in the form of open lectures and stalls (over 28) and is generally held in March.[15] Registration is free for students, but you must be a member of the Society. Royal Society of Medicine student membership costs around £25 and is about £65 per year for Young Fellows' membership (0–2 years since qualification, i.e. Foundation doctors).[16]

A successful Leicester University-based medical career fair went national for the first time in July 2006. The fair focuses on available specialties and medicine-related fields. Skills sessions, workshops and speeches occur throughout the two days. There is a small admission fee that covers attendance at all the available events. For more information visit the website www.medicalcareers.com.

Do not forget that finding sufficient information about different specialties is worth little if you do not know enough about yourself. You have to be able to match your talents and abilities with the options available, both clinical and non-clinical. Now that you know what career support and information you should be getting, and where you can go to find it, the rest is up to you.

References

1   Carnall D. Career guidance for doctors. *BMJ*. 1997; **315**: 6.

2   Allen I. *Doctors and Their Careers*. London: Policies Studies Institute; 1998.

3   Jackson C, Ball JE and Hirsh W et al. *Informing Choices: the need for career advice in medical training*. Cambridge: National Institute for Careers Education and Counselling; 2001.

4   BMA Board of Medical Education. *Signposting Medical Careers for Doctors*. London: BMA; 2003.

5   Modernising Medical Careers Working Group for Career Management. *Career Management: An Approach for Medical Schools, Deaneries, Royal Colleges and Trusts*. London: Department of Health; 2005.

6   www.mmc.nhs.uk/pages/careers

7   www.nhscareers.nhs.uk/home.html

8   www.medicalforum.com

9   Leung W and Birks K. Giving and seeking career guidance. *BMJ Career Focus*. 2001; **322**: 2.

10 Porter RW and Clayton B. Letters: career guidance for doctors. *BMJ*. 1998; **316**: 75.

11 Hutton-Taylor S. Do it yourself career guidance. *BMJ Careers*. 1996; **313**: 2.

12 Stern C. Career intentions of pre-registration house officers and the influence of career advice. *Br J Hosp Med*. 2005; **66**: 477–9.

13   www.pastest.co.uk
14   www.bmjcareersfair.com
15   www.rsm.ac.uk/students/studmeet.htm#march
16   www.rsm.ac.uk/membersh/submem.htm

Further reading

Bache J. Choosing a career. *BMJ Career Focus.* 1999; **318**: 2.

Gale R and Grant J. *Sci4 5. The Specialty Choice Inventory: computer-based careers advice for doctors in training.* Milton Keynes: Open University Centre for Education in Medicine; 2001.

Turya E. *Your Career after PLAB: surviving tools for young doctors.* Manchester: Edukon; 2003.

5

Mentors and educational supervisors

Mentors can be an invaluable source of support during medical school. Later in your career, as a Foundation doctor, you will also receive support from an educational supervisor. This chapter sets out the factors that comprise a 'perfect mentor', how to go about finding a mentor and the best case scenario of how mentors can be useful.

The British Medical Association (BMA) strongly advocates mentoring at all stages of medical education and throughout a doctor's career. In 2003, the BMA lobbied for the development of a mentoring system for all doctors and called on the government to resource it appropriately.[1] With increasing pressures on everyone's time, and the need to make career decisions earlier than previously, mentoring provides both personal and professional support allowing individuals to develop knowledge, skills, attributes and enhance their practice.[2]

What mentoring is

Mentoring has many definitions. The Department of Health (DoH) and the National Health Service (NHS) value mentoring, and after an inquiry, the Standing Committee on Postgraduate Medical Education (SCOPME) defined mentoring as a:

> ... process whereby an experienced, highly regarded empathetic person (the mentor), guides another individual (the mentee) in the development and re-examination of their own ideas, learning, and personal and professional development. The mentor, who often, but not necessarily works in the same organisation or field as the mentee, achieves this by listening and talking in confidence to the mentee.[3]

In the most recent *Modernising Medical Careers* (MMC) publication, mentoring is defined as:

> a relationship where one individual (the mentor) guides another to explore and expand on their own ideas, so that they learn and develop both personally and professionally.[4]

The list of definitions in both healthcare and organisation settings is extensive and they all sound rather similar. Collating the many and different explanations, the main elements which comprise mentoring include:[1,2,4,5,6,7]

- A professional relationship that should last over a fixed timescale, on a continuing basis and long term.
- Professional development, career progression and personal support:
  - mentoring should be a significant feature of an individual's career; especially at times of development, transitions and changes, for example between grades or placements
  - mentoring should help you to: take control of your career; understand how career choices are made and the wider socio-economic factors that may influence these choices; develop self-awareness and knowledge about your skills and abilities; investigate career pathways and opportunities and promote life-long learning throughout the career continuum
  - it should provide support to enable you to manage your own career by helping you develop effective career, life-planning and decision-making skills; this should occur through self-direction, personal control and responsibility.
- An opportunity to learn and develop whether your starting point is unsatisfactory or excellent.
- A mentor is generally a senior, experienced and respected member of the medical profession who can use their own experiences to guide the mentee to discuss, explore, develop, expand and later re-examine their own ideas and come to their own decisions. The mentee should not simply be told what to do.
- Issues should be explored in a constructive and non-threatening way.
- Mentor–mentee interaction should be confidential, so that the mentee can speak freely without fear of reprisal. Thus it should also be neutral and unbiased.
- Mentors and mentees should meet regularly, but not necessarily frequently.
- A mentor should be empathetic and someone who listens.
- Mentors and mentees need not be in the same organisation (and not in a direct management role with one another).

Educational supervisors

Educational supervisors are assigned to Foundation doctors, not medical students, and are concerned with helping you identify and meet your educational or training needs through a personal development plan.[5] The career support they provide is vital as they aid both career management and career education:

- *Career management* is a pro-active process entwined with career development. Your educational supervisor should guide you in how to manage your own career by helping you develop effective career, life-planning and decision-making skills through self-direction, personal control and responsibility throughout your career.[4]
- *Career education* occurs when educational supervisors help you to take control of your career by helping you to understand how career choices are made. This involves helping you to appreciate the wider socio-economic factors that may influence these choices, develop self-awareness and knowledge about your skills and abilities, investigate career pathways and opportunities, and promote life-long learning throughout your career.[4]

Some educational supervisors also provide career counselling and assist you in reflecting on and evaluating your career and life plans, especially at transitions in your life. Others may give practical or emotional support as well, but this is not really in their remit. If you cannot find a mentor who covers the whole scope of mentoring, but are assigned an educational supervisor, make use of them. Regular appraisal is a good way to boost your morale and your motivation, providing that you are performing well.

In the following sections the term 'mentor' is used to cover all mentoring roles. Therefore, when career development is discussed, this term also includes educational supervisors.

Why you should have a mentor[2]

Everyone tends to be stressed these days. You may have too much to do and not enough time. You do not always feel you can tell anyone in medicine how you really feel for fear of being seen as weak. However, things can be different. The mentoring relationship will give you the chance to share these feelings with someone in confidence, someone who has dealt with them before. It gives you the chance to explore your real thoughts, express your views, test out ideas and raise questions you may not have previously considered. A mentor will give you the opportunity to reflect, allowing you to work through your own issues using a combination of support and challenges without them attempting to solve the problems for you. In this supportive and confidential environment you can take a step back and look at yourself honestly in all the roles that you perform. With regards to your career you may have serious questions about where you are in your career, where you want to go next and how to get there.

Mentoring is a professional support mechanism. It provides you with a port of call if you are encountering any communication or relationship difficulties, are having difficulties coping with stress, need help to avoid using adverse coping strategies (such as drink or drugs) or if you believe you are facing burn-out.

Finally, mentoring is a dynamic process; with each mentor–mentee relationship usually lasting about a year. Individuals' requirements change throughout their career. Therefore mentoring can provide relevant and applicable guidance, ideas and advice at these junctures. This may also mean that at these different points in your career, you may need different mentors.

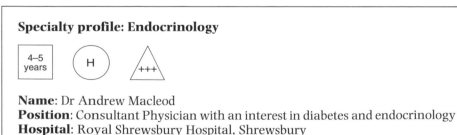

Specialty profile: Endocrinology

Name: Dr Andrew Macleod
Position: Consultant Physician with an interest in diabetes and endocrinology
Hospital: Royal Shrewsbury Hospital, Shrewsbury
Daily activities: I work full-time for the NHS (11 sessions) and also do a small amount of private practice. *Monday*: Endocrine clinic, with consultant colleague, SpR, SHO and endocrine nurse. Lunchtime: endocrine meeting. Ward round of acute admissions and occasional evening clinical meetings. *Tuesday*: Diabetes

clinic (general and young persons), with two clinical assistants; monthly neuropathy clinic. Lunchtime: diabetes meetings; teaching, admin, referrals. Occasional evening: Diabetes UK patient meetings. *Wednesday*: Monthly community clinic 34 miles away in Wales; well-supported with local GPs, community diabetes specialist nurse, chiropodists; looking at retinal photographs; radioiodine clinic. Lunchtime: 'grand round'; meetings; catch-up time; occasional ante-natal clinic. *Thursday*: Ward round with team; diabetes clinic at another hospital. *Friday*: Administration, referrals, planning, discussion with GPs, organisational work, meetings. I am a member of the diabetes and endocrine centre; there is always activity going on; chiropody, diabetes advice and education, retinal screening, dietetics, troubleshooting, endocrine tests, etc.

Qualities required: The ability to put oneself in the position of other people; working well within a team; reaching out into the community; planning whole services; reading the future!

Pros: Diabetes: Lots of patient contact; knowing most of the patients in the hospital and people in the Tesco superstore (possibly a con)! Good relationships within diabetes team; advantages of developing better service, close contact with the community and GPs; it is a common problem, so there are lots of people. Endocrinology: Good contrast to diabetes. Rare problems (apart from thyroid, etc.), less people! Fascinating: biochemistry in the human. Simple treatments usually do work and the patients usually get better.

Cons: Time pressure (always more to do with no time); pressure on clinics (patient overload, waiting times, etc.). Trying to organise community services can be frustrating. Trying to change patients' lifestyles.

Sub-specialties: Specialist endocrine services: mineral metabolism, adrenal disorders, pituitary disease, obesity, growth, endocrine in pregnancy; diabetes: young persons service, diabetes foot problems, diabetes/obstetric service, diabetic eye disease, impotence, renal/diabetes, neuropathy.

Allied specialties: Any general medical specialty; renal medicine; geriatrics; general practice. Attachment to Diabetes Centre offers exposure to clinics, specialist nurses, dieticians and podiatrists. GP diabetes clinics may also be helpful. Try some endocrinology. General medicine attachment linked to diabetes consultant.

Royal College website address: www.rcplondon.ac.uk

Benefits of mentoring

Mentoring is an essential component of career advice for both medical students and doctors. It has been identified as beneficial and advantageous as there is evidence of its positive effect in medicine.[6] The benefits of mentoring will invariably differ between individuals and different schemes. Such benefits are also difficult to quantify. However, the following possible benefits most associated with mentoring are listing under various headings below in Box 5.1.[1,2,4,7,8]

Box 5.1:   Benefits of mentoring

Workplace benefits:

- Improved work performance
- Improved relationships and communication, including an increased sense of collegiality
- Improved retention rates and job satisfaction

Acquisition of new or improvement of existing skills:

- Regained and/or increased confidence in taking action, taking the lead, being yourself and dealing with difficult job situations or relationships
- Enhanced problem-solving and analytical skills
- Ability to overcome setbacks, obstacles and change positively
- Leads to an open and flexible attitude to learning
- Develop new ways to approach and manage problems
- Ability to improve the identification of core problems and to understand the underlying issues
- Increased skills at influencing interpersonal relationships
- Encourages reflective practice and self-knowledge
- Develops effective career and life planning and decision-making skills

Improved learning opportunities:

- Scope for new ideas, new insights to perspectives and ways of managing problems, situations or your career
- Provides learning opportunities which increase knowledge and skills, including technical skills and help with new tasks
- Identifies specific educational needs
- Enhanced learning through learned reflective practice
- Provides advice and skills about how to manage people
- Increased political knowledge, developed sense of values and ethical perspective, as well as an overall greater understanding of the perspective of others

Career benefits:

- Opportunity for new ideas, insights, perspectives and ways of managing your career by pro-active exploration and decision-making about all possible career options
- Support to enable you to manage your own career through self-direction, personal control and responsibility

---

- Encourages reflective and evaluative thinking about your career and life plans (especially during transitions and life changes, or if you experience particular career difficulties)
- Provides in-depth focus and support when making career decisions, either before or during your career
- Facilitates your career education (understand how career choices are made, the wider socio-economic factors that may influence these choices and how to investigate career pathways and opportunities)
- Promotes life-long learning throughout the career continuum
- Possibly some degree of sponsorship and recommendation from the mentor, and access to the mentor's informal network

Benefits of self-discovery:

- Increased sense of well-being
- A clearer understanding of yourself
- Encourages self-awareness and empowerment
- Develop self-awareness (personality, academic ability, personal attributes) and knowledge about your skills and abilities

Mentoring can also be utilised to help support and promote cultural diversity or address issues of discrimination. Female consultants can provide mentoring to female junior doctors. Mentors from the same minority group as mentees can act as role models.

Traditionally, doctors have shown reluctance towards taking up mentoring schemes. Although this may be due to time constraints, it has been suggested that actively engaging in mentoring is seen as a weakness.[9] The potential advantages of mentoring need to be highlighted, with a wider range of information offered, in terms of the potential benefits and limitations of participation, so more medical students and doctors are willing to participate. 'Mentoring should be promoted as a positive and active method to enhance one's career.'[1]

Finding a mentor

When postgraduate deaneries were contacted to explore the range of mentoring schemes that are available it became apparent that there is a vast difference in such schemes between the various deaneries.[1]

In some deaneries, mentoring is part of the remit assigned to trusts and is not centrally co-ordinated (Eastern Deanery, South Western Deanery). Many ad hoc mentoring projects also exist (North of Scotland, Oxford). Most mentoring schemes co-ordinated by deaneries were often targeted at consultants (Scotland, West Midlands, Wessex, Oxford), whereas other schemes focused on overseas and international doctors (Manchester) or refugee and asylum-seeking doctors (West of Scotland). Other postgraduate deaneries offered peer-mentoring schemes, a counselling service or did not offer a scheme but were able to refer doctors to relevant schemes. Other mentoring schemes can be found through medical schools, royal colleges or individual trusts or departments. More recently, schemes have been designed to encourage a similar developmental relationship between peers.

So what situation are you in?

- You are already in a mentoring scheme. If this is so, use this chapter to maximise that experience. Make a list of objectives, if you have not done so yet, and go through all the different ways a mentor can be utilised. You should also evaluate your mentor–mentee relationship to date to see if it is working for you (*see below*).
- You do not have a mentor assigned to you.[2] You really should start doing some research into schemes that may include you, as the benefits of having a mentor are far-reaching.

Does your university, hospital trust or library have a list of individuals who are willing to be mentors? If not, is there anyone you know who has been a mentor before, or could fulfil the mentoring criteria? What sort of person do you need (*see below*)? In a survey of BMA members, consisting of doctors and medical students, 54% of respondents said they would go to senior doctors for advice, 21% would go to lecturers, trainers or tutors, and 6% said they would go to people in supervisory roles.[10]

When you have a shortlist, go and meet the individuals. Find out if they would be willing, and able, to commit to a voluntary mentor–mentee relationship. They must have the time and be enthusiastic about taking on the role. If they do not know about mentoring, find out what they think it entails, and take this *Handbook* with you!

See if you are able to build a rapport with your chosen mentor. Not only should it be someone with whom you would work well, they should be able to challenge you and make you think from different perspectives.

Ask if they have any previous experience of being a mentor, or indeed a mentee. Ask them how it went, what they can offer and about the opportunities for both of you.

At different points in your career, you may need different mentors. Not only that, but you may opt to have different mentors at the same time. You may want more than one mentor at a time if they have different qualities, personalities or experiences, and can thus support you in different ways or for different aspects of either your personal or working life, or in your career.

A mentor can be any suitably experienced medical, allied health or non-medical professional and does not need to be in a managerial role in the same organisation as you.

The qualities of a good mentor

Traditionally, a mentor is an older and wiser colleague who can use their knowledge, skills and experience to empower the mentee. Before using any criteria as a checklist to find your perfect mentor, why not think carefully and ask yourself a few questions.

- What personality traits do I possess? This may be a good time to look back to the personality section of Chapter 3.
- What strengths and weaknesses do I have that may need support? Use the personality section of Chapter 3 and the forms in Appendix 2 and Appendix 3.
- What type of person can provide the type of support you have identified? The personality toolkit in Chapter 3 may help with this.
- What type of people do I get on well with? Ask yourself which type would challenge you with a different, broader and more diverse perspective than your own.
- What do I actually want to get from this mentor–mentee relationship?
- What kind of person will be able to help me achieve this?
- What qualities would I like them to possess?

Someone who has been a mentor before would be ideal as they should be well aware of how the relationship works. What is certain is that a degree of research is going to be needed before you find the right mentor for you, but it will be worth it in the end.

Specialty profile: Forensic psychiatry

| 5 years | M | ++ |

Name: Dr Anne Aboaja
Position: Specialist Registrar in Forensic Psychiatry
Hospital: Arnold Lodge, Leicester
Daily activities: Mornings: communication meeting, ward round or clinical ward work; assessment for court reports or referrals; meetings. Lunchtimes: academic meeting with case presentation or journal club. Afternoons: out-patient clinic at local prison; tribunal; dictating a report or clinical ward work; educational supervision with consultant.
Qualities required: Good oral and written communication skills; non-judgemental approach; ability to work in a team; psychodynamically minded; clear thinker and decisive; empathic; reflective.
Pros: Holistic approach to patient care with the required resources; time to take a thorough history and offer a management plan; helping some of the most socially disadvantaged patients in the NHS; trying to understand the relationship between mental illness and crime; going to court; caring for both mental and physical health; the legal aspects (for example, case law, Mental Health Act, criminal justice system); interesting medicine (for example, treatment-resistant schizophrenia, temporal lobe epilepsy, substance misuse).
Cons: Have to produce long reports; relatively slow admission and discharge rate.
Sub-specialties: Adolescent forensic psychiatry; learning disabilities forensic psychiatry; mental illness forensic psychiatry; women's forensic psychiatry; personality disorder forensic psychiatry; forensic psychotherapy.
Allied specialties: Drugs and alcohol; psychotherapy; general adult psychiatry; rehabilitation psychiatry. Insight into general psychiatry can also be gained in any psychiatric specialty plus some voluntary services such as Nightline. Also getting experience of prison medicine or substance misuse services will help you.
Royal College website address: www.rcpsych.ac.uk

Box 5.2 contains lists of both essential and desirable qualities to look for in a mentor, as described in *The Good Mentoring Toolkit for Healthcare*.[2]

Box 5.2:   Qualities to look for in a mentor

Essential qualities

Impartial	Respectful	Ethical
Good listener	Effective leader	Supportive
Skilled in feedback	Interested	Non-judgemental
Perceptive	Able to challenge	Self-aware
Trustworthy	Chemistry (intellectual and emotional compatibility)	

Desirable qualities

Knowledge	Technical expertise	Instructor
Authority	Adviser	Seniority
Inspiring	Knows the health service	Experience
Patient	Able to receive feedback	

How to make the most of your mentor[2]

Discuss the terms of your mentoring partnership before commencing the relationship. By setting clear aims and objectives both of you will know what is expected and what needs to be achieved. These will not be the same for every person, or throughout their career, as each individual will have diverse requirements that will vary at different points in their career. This initial understanding will allow for a more successful and fulfilling mentor–mentee relationship.

First, set objectives covering the main purpose and focus of your meetings. Think about what you want to achieve in these sessions. For example, if you want to focus on career development you may want to answer the following questions.

- What is my ideal job?
- How do I get there?
- Do my skills and attributes suit this discipline?
- Do I want to tackle work-related issues, political issues, leadership styles, networking opportunities?

You should discuss the questions you have with your mentor and then plan when and how you want to cover them. This is a personal development plan. Think about whether you want to leave a set amount of time each session to discuss new issues. Prepare thoroughly for each session in order to get the most out of it.

Once you have a set agenda, create ground rules as to:

- where, when and for how long you will meet each time
- the length of time the relationship will last
- when you will have reviews to re-assess the contract and how you will evaluate the relationship
- who will arrange the meetings
- if and how you will record the meetings and who keeps these records

- what to do if either party needs to cancel and how many cancellations will occur before the contract is reviewed
- what to do if either mentor or mentee wants to opt out of the contract
- confidentiality and any exceptions
- personal boundaries or any potential conflicts of interest
- both the mentor and the mentee should be aware that the mentee's autonomy must be respected; that is, you can choose to follow or ignore any guidance given (it is guidance, not instruction)[11]
- suggest other sources of information or appropriate advisers.

Brief your mentor with your career aims, achievements to date, perceived weaknesses and strengths, and the nature of any advice sought in this area. This allows the mentor to research into any relevant issues or refer you to a more appropriate person if needs be.[10]

Evaluating your mentor–mentee partnership

Mentoring relationships, and schemes in general, can only be improved through evaluating feedback and monitoring schemes. While setting your ground rules you should decide when your contract review will take place. It is imperative that you keep to this in order to maintain the efficacy of the relationship.

During the review certain questions must be asked.[2]

- Are the sessions following the mentee's agenda, sticking to the time limits and issues in question?
- Have there been any cancellations? By whom, and why? What needs to be done about this?
- Is the relationship working? What are the strengths in the relationship and what needs to be worked on?
- Is the appropriate amount of challenging occurring? Is the correct amount of listening, support and information also occurring?
- Do you feel you are acquiring new knowledge and skills, developing personally and professionally? Are these being transferred to your working environment?

Lack of time and poorly matched pairs are the most common problems encountered in mentoring schemes.[1] Other common pitfalls include under- or over-management, poor objective setting and preparation, too little or too much formality, and breach of confidentiality.[2] If any of these problems become an issue they must be tackled head on. Review your rules and clarify or re-write them so that they are more realistic and achievable.

Mentoring is extremely beneficial to an individual when matched with a compatible mentor. There are ongoing debates as to whether or not mentoring schemes should be voluntary or compulsory. Although mentoring has immense benefits, making the scheme compulsory has potential adverse effects.[1] Regular feedback from mentees is essential to monitor and evaluate schemes, and in order to improve and sustain the level of quality of mentoring schemes.

Publicity is needed to advertise the positive benefits of mentoring schemes. Although lack of time is a big problem for everyone these days, potential mentees must realise that being involved in mentoring is a pertinent use of their time. Publicity is especially needed to destroy myths that mentoring is for the weak and needy, and that confidentiality is not respected. Some of you may never have even thought about mentoring or how you might go about arranging it, but perhaps now you have a much better idea and realise that mentoring is an important part in the life-long learning of doctors.

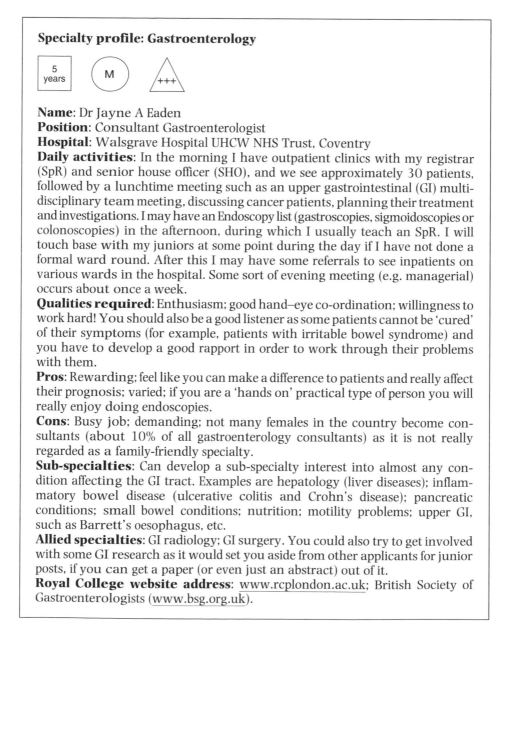

Specialty profile: Gastroenterology

Name: Dr Jayne A Eaden
Position: Consultant Gastroenterologist
Hospital: Walsgrave Hospital UHCW NHS Trust, Coventry
Daily activities: In the morning I have outpatient clinics with my registrar (SpR) and senior house officer (SHO), and we see approximately 30 patients, followed by a lunchtime meeting such as an upper gastrointestinal (GI) multi-disciplinary team meeting, discussing cancer patients, planning their treatment and investigations. I may have an Endoscopy list (gastroscopies, sigmoidoscopies or colonoscopies) in the afternoon, during which I usually teach an SpR. I will touch base with my juniors at some point during the day if I have not done a formal ward round. After this I may have some referrals to see inpatients on various wards in the hospital. Some sort of evening meeting (e.g. managerial) occurs about once a week.
Qualities required: Enthusiasm; good hand–eye co-ordination; willingness to work hard! You should also be a good listener as some patients cannot be 'cured' of their symptoms (for example, patients with irritable bowel syndrome) and you have to develop a good rapport in order to work through their problems with them.
Pros: Rewarding; feel like you can make a difference to patients and really affect their prognosis; varied; if you are a 'hands on' practical type of person you will really enjoy doing endoscopies.
Cons: Busy job; demanding; not many females in the country become consultants (about 10% of all gastroenterology consultants) as it is not really regarded as a family-friendly specialty.
Sub-specialties: Can develop a sub-specialty interest into almost any condition affecting the GI tract. Examples are hepatology (liver diseases); inflammatory bowel disease (ulcerative colitis and Crohn's disease); pancreatic conditions; small bowel conditions; nutrition; motility problems; upper GI, such as Barrett's oesophagus, etc.
Allied specialties: GI radiology; GI surgery. You could also try to get involved with some GI research as it would set you aside from other applicants for junior posts, if you can get a paper (or even just an abstract) out of it.
Royal College website address: www.rcplondon.ac.uk; British Society of Gastroenterologists (www.bsg.org.uk).

References

1 British Medical Association. *Exploring Mentoring*. London: BMA Board of Medical Education; 2004.

2 Bayley H, Chambers R and Donovan C. *The Good Mentoring Toolkit for Healthcare*. Oxford: Radcliffe Publishing; 2004.

3 Standing Committee on Postgraduate Medical and Dental Education. *Supporting Doctors and Dentists at Work: an enquiry into mentoring*. London: SCOPME; 1998.

4 Modernising Medical Careers Working Group for Career Management. *Career Management: An Approach for Medical Schools, Deaneries, Royal Colleges and Trusts*. London: Department of Health; 2005.

5 Chambers R. *Survival Skills for GPs*. Oxford: Radcliffe Medical Press; 1999.

6 Connor MP, Bynoe AG and Redfern N et al. Developing senior doctors as mentors: a form of continuing professional development. *Med Ed*. 2000; **34**: 745–53.

7 Incomes Data Services.*Personnel Policy and Practice: mentoring*. Surrey: Unwin Brothers/ The Gresham Press; 2000.

8 Oxley J and Fleming B. *Mentoring for Doctors: signposts to current practice for career grade doctors*. London: Department of Health; 2004.

9 Snell J. Head to head. *Health Service Journal*. 1999; **109**: 22–5.

10 Jackson C, Ball JE and Hirsh W et al. *Informing Choices: the need for career advice in medical training*. Cambridge: National Institute for Careers Education and Counselling; 2001.

11 Leung W amd Birks K. Giving and seeking career guidance. *BMJ Career Focus*. 2001; **322**: 2.

6

Broadening your clinical experience

The medical school curriculum is designed so that you can choose what you want to study at certain times. This chapter highlights the parts of your course that give you the freedom to decide what you want to study and how you can make best use of these times.

Broadening your clinical experience with focused placements has the potential to support you in making informed and appropriate decisions about your career development early on in your training.[1] The best way to decide whether or not you enjoy a particular aspect of medicine is to experience it first hand. There are many opportunities to sample various aspects of medicine within your course, including student-selected components, your elective and intercalated degrees (where available and should you choose to do one). Other opportunities also exist outside your course, such as part-time jobs, summer jobs, work experience and specialty courses. During your Foundation years some deaneries also allow you to sample additional career alternatives 'tasters' in other areas of medicine for a few days at a time. However, you may have to use your study leave entitlement to do this. You will have to write a report on your time in that specialty which includes the skills that would be required in addition to the ones you possess to succeed in that specialty.

You may want to use these optional components of your curriculum to do the following.

- Fill in the deficiencies in your course as well as learning about the subjects inadequately covered to address your learning needs. For example, many medical courses do not allow time for specialist areas such as ear, nose and throat (ENT), ophthalmology, dermatology or A&E, and you may wish to use your time to sample them.
- Broaden areas of interest that can apply to any career, such as academic placements and other areas you may wish to know more about.
- Follow any particular interests (but try to remain open-minded).

Student-selected components

Student-selected components (SSCs), or student-selected modules (SSMs) as they are known in some universities, were created in 1993 following the General Medical Council (GMC) publication *Tomorrow's Doctors*,[2] which recommended that students should be allowed to follow their own interests beyond the curriculum. SSCs were designed to allow students to study a particular area of interest in more depth. Some medical schools allow you to take one or more SSC abroad as well as your elective. You could pursue new interests, develop existing ones or provide experience that is relevant to the preceding, or a future, main module:

> 'I chose an SSC module in A&E at the Royal Shrewsbury Hospital. It was a great chance to develop my basic skills, gain confidence in speaking and eliciting histories, as well as developing an understanding of symptom differentials. This attachment also allowed me to become independent in my thinking with respect to investigations and management of patients. I saw a variety of medicine and was able to develop and further my knowledge.' (Janaki Gnananandha, third-year medical student, Keele University)

Medical schools devote markedly different portions of the course to SSCs, which can encompass between two and five weeks at different points throughout your medical studies from Year 1 onwards. SSCs in the clinical years usually become more clinically oriented and self-directed.[3]

SSCs can be medical, clinical, managerial, a project or research-based. They can also be non-medical but remain medically related. These include the history of medicine, medicine art, modern languages, music or sign language, complementary and alternative medicine, sports medicine, radiology, journalism, arts or humanities. You could also choose to work with the police, take part in scientific and community projects (Manchester), become involved in medical publishing (Oxford) or study shiatsu and yoga (Peninsula). The possibilities are endless. Although a list of options and placements is often held by the university, now that you have read about the many different types of SSC on offer, how about proposing your own?

Students are usually allocated places on a one-to-one or a two-to-one basis to a consultant supervisor. How the student spends that time is entirely for negotiation between student and supervisor. It is worth noting that, apart from your own personal aims and learning objectives for the SSC, your university may have others in mind for each of these aspects of your course. For example, at East Anglia the aims of SSCs fall into two parts:[3]

- To assess a student's ability to gather, appraise and present information within a set list of domains.
- To learn how to review and appraise research papers, assessed through a formal written appraisal for every unit.

Thus, SSCs may test a student's ability to:[4]

- gather data by questionnaire and/or oral interview
- use library and information services to perform literature searches
- gather data from the literature and critically evaluate it as well as ranking the range and level of authority of different forms of scientific literature
- compile information into a written report that addresses the topic to be investigated
- use computer technology to compile and submit a written report and be able to deliver an oral presentation.

Other learning objectives may include how you demonstrate:[4]

- achievement of the specific objectives originally set
- appreciation of the legal and personal needs to respect confidentiality and/or sensitive issues relating to human subjects
- reflection of how you have worked with other healthcare professionals

- in-depth knowledge of one particular subject including, if appropriate, public health aspects, prevention, epidemiology, treatment options and future development in relation to one or more patients.

The best thing you can do at the start of your SSC is to determine what objectives you and your university are setting so that you know how to meet them.

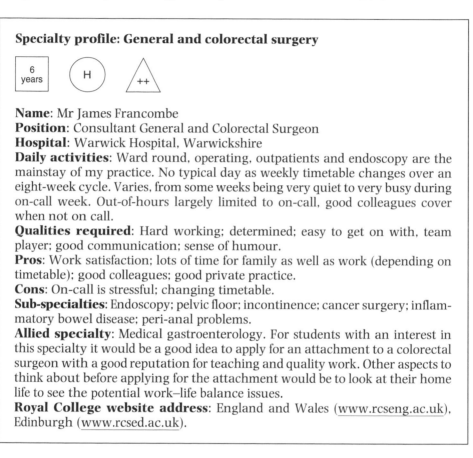

Specialty profile: General and colorectal surgery

Name: Mr James Francombe
Position: Consultant General and Colorectal Surgeon
Hospital: Warwick Hospital, Warwickshire
Daily activities: Ward round, operating, outpatients and endoscopy are the mainstay of my practice. No typical day as weekly timetable changes over an eight-week cycle. Varies, from some weeks being very quiet to very busy during on-call week. Out-of-hours largely limited to on-call, good colleagues cover when not on call.
Qualities required: Hard working; determined; easy to get on with, team player; good communication; sense of humour.
Pros: Work satisfaction; lots of time for family as well as work (depending on timetable); good colleagues; good private practice.
Cons: On-call is stressful; changing timetable.
Sub-specialties: Endoscopy; pelvic floor; incontinence; cancer surgery; inflammatory bowel disease; peri-anal problems.
Allied specialty: Medical gastroenterology. For students with an interest in this specialty it would be a good idea to apply for an attachment to a colorectal surgeon with a good reputation for teaching and quality work. Other aspects to think about before applying for the attachment would be to look at their home life to see the potential work–life balance issues.
Royal College website address: England and Wales (www.rcseng.ac.uk), Edinburgh (www.rcsed.ac.uk).

Your assessment will include your written report of the case, the oral presentation, workbook, poster presentation or written examination. Your attendance is also taken into account as well as your performance against the learning objectives agreed between yourself and your supervisor.

In the article 'Getting the most out of your SSMs',[5] students were asked about their opinions and experiences of SSCs. Some sensible top tips were:

- start early
- read information carefully and e-mail tutors to clarify details
- think about how much time you want to, or can, give a placement
- only request choices you want
- do not be put off by people attempting to stop you doing what you want
- do something you will enjoy, which will also further your medical education

- find a tutor who shares your special interest – the more interested your tutor is and the more interested you are the more you will gain from completing the SSC
- do something original
- go into your SSC with an open mind
- do not be disheartened; your fifth choice could be just as rewarding – you will often find, even if you have not been given your first-choice SSC, that so long as you 'get into' your project you will probably end up enjoying it
- do not waste it.

Elective

The elective is an integral part of the medical course and is usually a period of between 8 and 12 weeks taken as a continuous block of study. It is often seen as a major highlight of the time spent at medical school.

The timing of the elective depends on the university, but it is usually scheduled during clinical studies so that you already have a good broad base in order to maximise your learning. It is an invaluable learning resource and not a holiday, though a holiday can be, and often is, added on.

Think what you want to achieve

'I did my elective at St John's Medical College Hospital in Bangalore, India. I chose this as it is a charity and privately run hospital in a large city in India, and I saw the elective as an opportunity to throw myself into a completely different culture in a country I knew very little about yet which is rich in diversity in terms of places to visit and the people that live there. From my experience, I learnt that very different factors influence healthcare in India compared to the UK, largely religion and costs! I also had the opportunity to explore cities, mountains, national parks and beaches – experiencing the Hindi culture and Indian way of life at first hand. All in all, an amazing eight weeks.' (Gemma Cooper-Hobson, final-year medical student at Manchester University [Keele cohort])

As it is a period of own self-directed learning, many students choose to go overseas, taking the chance to see non-National Health Service (NHS) medicine and to experience the practice of medicine in an unfamiliar setting where the scientific, social, economic or cultural standards are different. There are very diverse healthcare systems across the globe, from the underdeveloped third-world hospitals where you may get a lot of 'hands on' experience, to the ultra modern and high-tech institutes where you may see ground-breaking procedures. Or, instead of practising your clinical skills, how about electing to teach in Tanzania, like four medical students from University College London did?[6] The opportunities are endless; depending on your learning needs, interests and what you want to achieve. It is what you make of it.

Research, research, research

You have to organise your elective yourself, which means you can apply wherever you wish. Unfortunately, there are scams out there so be careful if money is being asked for in advance. Make sure your supervisor is medically qualified and that you are not putting yourself at undue risk. Also make sure you start planning your elective early. The most popular electives are often taken up years in advance and the application procedure for some electives can be extremely complex and time-consuming. In view of current political instability in some areas, you should be aware of the safety issues and check about countries you intend to visit on the Foreign & Commonwealth Office website (www.fco.gov.uk/travel). You should recheck this advice just before leaving for your elective as political situations can change rapidly. The elective co-ordinators at your medical school will help if you have to change your plans suddenly because of such an event.

There are a lot of resources which provide information on electives to help with your choices. *The Medic's Guide to Work and Electives Around the World*[7] is a very user-friendly and informative manual. If you prefer information in a web-based form www.medicstravel.co.uk is a phenomenal resource and, through its connections with hundreds of hospitals across the globe, can arrange your elective for a £30 admin-istration fee. There is also the electives network,[8] which is available free to student members of the Medical Defence Union and has a database of over 110 country profiles with information on funding, flights, vaccinations and visas, and more than 4000 possible hospitals to apply to.

Speak to others

Some universities may provide a copy of addresses used by students in previous years, may have existing arrangements with international institutions, or may have student-led exchange programmes. For example, Guy's, King's and St Thomas' medical schools have special links with the Johns Hopkins University in the USA, the University of Hong Kong, the University of West Indies and the Moscow Medical Academy. Speak to previous elective students, doctors and consultants on the wards, and find out what they did and what they would not do now. Some universities also keep elective reports.

Be prepared

Make sure when choosing a place, you research the health and working conditions there. For information on infectious diseases you can go to www.doh.gov.uk/traveladvice. Sort out your vaccinations and HIV prophylaxis well in advance; there should be contacts at your medical school who can advise you on these. You should also make sure that your travel insurance covers you. There are some travel insurance policies specifically for medical students on their elective. It is worth researching these. Accommodation may be arranged for you, but you must check this is the case. Extra bursaries are available to help with this (*see* 'Money matters' below).

Important information about travel arrangements

Some students have found themselves in trouble on their elective. If you are going abroad check the expiry date on your passport, as some countries require you to have at least six months left at the date of your return.

Check whether you need a visa and if you do, ensure it is the correct one. Allow plenty of time for this to be processed. The Foreign & Commonwealth Office website travel advice section provides useful advice on visas and other requirements.

You will not require a work permit visa, as you are not being paid and you do not usually require a student study visa, hence, you should apply for a normal visitor's visa unless your host university or hospital instructs you otherwise. Always check with them before setting off on your travels.

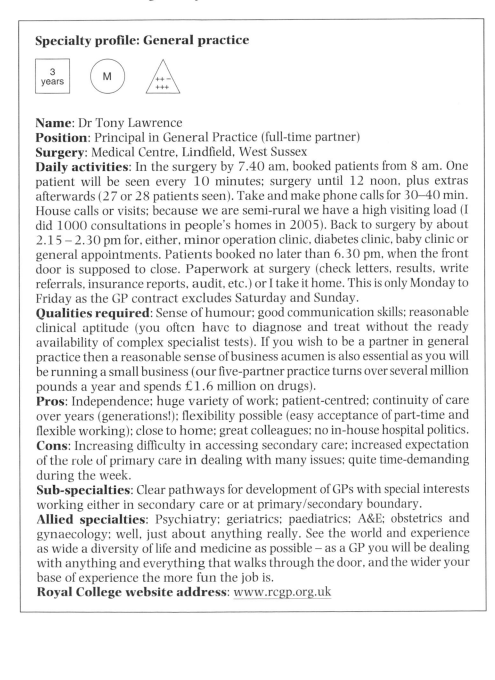

Specialty profile: General practice

Name: Dr Tony Lawrence
Position: Principal in General Practice (full-time partner)
Surgery: Medical Centre, Lindfield, West Sussex
Daily activities: In the surgery by 7.40 am, booked patients from 8 am. One patient will be seen every 10 minutes; surgery until 12 noon, plus extras afterwards (27 or 28 patients seen). Take and make phone calls for 30–40 min. House calls or visits; because we are semi-rural we have a high visiting load (I did 1000 consultations in people's homes in 2005). Back to surgery by about 2.15 – 2.30 pm for, either, minor operation clinic, diabetes clinic, baby clinic or general appointments. Patients booked no later than 6.30 pm, when the front door is supposed to close. Paperwork at surgery (check letters, results, write referrals, insurance reports, audit, etc.) or I take it home. This is only Monday to Friday as the GP contract excludes Saturday and Sunday.
Qualities required: Sense of humour; good communication skills; reasonable clinical aptitude (you often have to diagnose and treat without the ready availability of complex specialist tests). If you wish to be a partner in general practice then a reasonable sense of business acumen is also essential as you will be running a small business (our five-partner practice turns over several million pounds a year and spends £1.6 million on drugs).
Pros: Independence; huge variety of work; patient-centred; continuity of care over years (generations!); flexibility possible (easy acceptance of part-time and flexible working); close to home; great colleagues; no in-house hospital politics.
Cons: Increasing difficulty in accessing secondary care; increased expectation of the role of primary care in dealing with many issues; quite time-demanding during the week.
Sub-specialties: Clear pathways for development of GPs with special interests working either in secondary care or at primary/secondary boundary.
Allied specialties: Psychiatry; geriatrics; paediatrics; A&E; obstetrics and gynaecology; well, just about anything really. See the world and experience as wide a diversity of life and medicine as possible – as a GP you will be dealing with anything and everything that walks through the door, and the wider your base of experience the more fun the job is.
Royal College website address: www.rcgp.org.uk

Insurance and malpractice cover

Universities usually do *not* insure you against malpractice and for health cover whilst you are on your elective. Contact the Medical Defence Union (MDU), Medical and Dental Defence Union of Scotland (MDDUS), Medical Protection Society (MPS) or any other medical defence organisation, to arrange insurance cover when travelling abroad on your elective.

If you are applying to North America, Canada or Israel you must enquire about malpractice cover. The MPS, MDU and MDDUS (free abroad) will help in the USA. The host university may make arrangements for you or the host university may direct you as to how you can obtain it. You will almost certainly have to pay for insurance cover in North America and the amounts vary. In Canada and Israel insurance is usually arranged for you but again you will have to pay.

The MDU has produced a useful guide on your elective placement, including malpractice cover. There is more information about medical defence organisations in the section on the roles of important organisations and societies.

Letters of recommendation

Letters of recommendation are not routinely provided for applicants for electives. However, if a letter of recommendation, or a letter to confirm your status as a student, is required in your individual case your medical school should provide one. Contact your medical school in good time to allow for administration.

After you have arranged it

Your university will probably require you to provide details of your elective, which may have to be on specific forms. Enquire at your own medical school with regard to what the procedure is.

Money matters

Unfortunately, you will have to find the funding for your elective yourself. Electives can be expensive, though it really does depend on what you want to do. There are numerous grants, awards (up to £600 from MDDUS), research awards, sponsorships, bursaries and prizes (you can win up to £1500 from the MDU) available. If you are well-organised you can get a considerable amount of support, although it is easier if you are incorporating some research into your elective, as most awards and grants are awarded in exchange for some sort of project report or research work. Grants and awards are sometimes offered as part of a competition, particularly if the elective is related to the professional body or organisation offering the money. For example, the Wellcome Trust offers a special research elective bursary. The BMA holds a list of organisations to which you can apply for funding. Information on research and development funding can also be found at www.rdinfo.org.uk. Currently, the database holds information from more than 1300 funding bodies, offering over 5000 different awards.

And now for something different

If you decide to stay in the same country as your medical school, do something useful or different with your time. How about getting involved in medical politics, a project at an academic or a pharmaceutical research centre or even working with the team doctor at a football club? Remember some of your peers, with whom you will be competing for Foundation places in the near future, will be off working with Tibetan monks in Lhasa's community hospital[9] or in the Gambia assisting a voluntary service overseas' paediatrician.[10] So try to be original and find something interesting and stimulating to do in your home country.

Intercalated degrees

Intercalated degrees[3] are usually one-year degree courses that can be undertaken during a year away from your medical degree in a variety of subjects related to medicine, and they provide an opportunity to pursue further study in an area of interest. In some universities students are allowed to study for the extra degree within other faculties of the university or at other institutes or universities. Consider doing this if you have a particular interest that cannot be fulfilled at your medical school, if your interest is in a very popular and oversubscribed subject, or if a particular university is renowned for a research interest that appeals to you.[9]

Interest in intercalated degrees has grown over the years as they allow you to study a particular area of interest in greater depth. They enable you to gain valuable skills in either clinical, laboratory or epidemiological research.[11]

You can obtain a Bachelor of Science (BSc), Bachelor of Medical Science (BMedSci), Bachelor of Arts (BA) or you can do a Masters in Medical Science (MMedSc) for an additional year of study. Such degrees are commonly undertaken once you have completed at least two years of study as a medical student, hence, after Year 2 or Year 3, though entry policies differ at different universities.

Traditionally, in some institutions, intercalated degrees were only open to high flyers. You would have had to have passed all your exams and not repeated a year, to be considered. Currently, in the Dundee School of Medicine, allocation is by invitation only but this is slowly changing. Allocation, however, may still be on a competitive basis, for example at Bart's and the London Queen Mary's School of Medicine. In other universities intercalated degrees are not only open to any student, but actively encouraged, such as in Bristol Medical School. Figures show that between 20% and 40% of medical students intercalate.[9] In medical schools where intercalated degrees are voluntary, as many as 50% of each year group intercalate at some point in their studies.[3] At some universities intercalating degrees are compulsory (e.g. the University of Nottingham).

Degrees may be awarded in research- or library-based projects. They can be medical as well as social science degrees. Biological sciences subjects you may be able to study include anthropology, psychology, anatomy, biochemistry, cell biology, physiology, microbiology, pharmacology, medical or molecular genetics, neuroscience, pathology, laboratory-based research project, sports medicine, forensic archaeology or even space physiology (Royal Free and University College Medical School). Degrees in integrated health science subjects are fewer in number and include public health, ethics and law, behavioural science, history of medicine as well as management (Imperial College School of Medicine).

The main consideration in extending the already lengthy medical course is that you will need to finance 12 additional months. Fees may be payable for the year but in some institutes separate funding may be available. At some universities tuition fees for this year are paid but you need to pay living costs. Find out about this before embarking on such a degree.

Intercalated degrees are thought to result in better study habits with higher 'deep' and 'strategic' learning scores.[12] They are also thought to be particularly useful if you are considering a career in research or academic medicine or teaching as a career. It is an opportunity to derive potentially publishable original research project material and have chance to publish papers, which adds weight to your CV.[13]

European exchange programmes

The International Federation of Medical Students' Association (IFMSA) is an international exchange scheme that allows medical students from across the world to literally swap places for a few weeks. This allows them to complete a clinical attachment in a range of countries. The exchange scheme is huge and involves over 100 countries. In Europe, the scheme involves Malta, Italy, Estonia and Germany. It costs the student £150 and they must provide their room for the exchange student while they are away.[5]

The European Community Action Scheme for the Mobility of University Students (Erasmus) was set up in 1987. It provides organisation and funding to enable university students of any discipline to take part in an exchange with another European country during part of their course.[14] In the minority of medical schools, these schemes allow you to study a foreign language and complete a period of study abroad. You usually spend up to three months (although it could be up to a year depending on the university) at various places in Europe, including France, Germany and Scandinavia. The exact amount of time, year of placement and location depend on your university and the links that it has in place; practices vary considerably between universities. There is also less emphasis on practising clinical medicine than there is with the elective.

Summer jobs, part-time work, work experience[3]

As well as casual work in bars and restaurants carried out by students of other subjects, many medical students choose to work as healthcare assistants, medical secretaries in hospitals or note summarisers in general practices. This work can usually be arranged through the teaching hospital, other local hospitals or via the GPs that take medical students on attachments, all of which would be on file at your medical school. There are also nursing agencies or nurse banks that you can sign up to directly.

Specialty profile: Genitourinary medicine

| 5 years | L | + – ++ |

Name: Dr Mike Walzman
Position: GUM Consultant
Hospital: George Eliot Hospital, Nuneaton
Daily activities: The specialty is primarily outpatient-based. I spend time within the Department on a daily basis doing at least one clinic session per day and sometimes an evening clinic too. The clinical spectrum ranges from sexual health check-ups, diagnosis and management of common sexually transmitted conditions and genital dermatological conditions, to the management of HIV-positive patients. On occasions, I am involved in inpatient management; usually of HIV-positive patients. Apart from doing clinics I have sessions for patient administration, teaching and my own continuing professional development.
Qualities required: Good communication; non-judgemental attitude; ability to put people at ease; good sense of humour!
Pros: The strong team spirit; large and important public health element to the job; dealing primarily with young, healthy patients; often able to give instant reassurance or very quick diagnoses and treatment; do not often have patients die; on-call commitments are usually either negligible or not too arduous; scope to develop a number of 'special interests' within the specialty; as it is a relatively small specialty most consultants will know each other.
Cons: The stigma attached to attending a GUM clinic, which can 'rub-off' onto those working within the specialty; however, nowadays, there is very little stigmatisation, patients in general feel comfortable about their attendance and I find that GUM health professionals are in fact highly regarded by colleagues; not generally a specialty for those who are hoping for private practice.
Sub-specialties: HIV; sexual dysfunction; genital dermatology/vulval disorders; psychosexual/psychotherapy. (Apart from HIV, the others would normally be for a special interest clinic and not form a major weekly commitment.)
Allied specialty: Infectious diseases; gynaecology; family planning; dermatology; immunology; virology; microbiology. Student should aim to spend more time (1–2 full weeks) in GUM with some time in one or more of the other sub-specialties.
Royal College website address: www.rcplondon.ac.uk; British Association for Sexual Health and HIV (www.bashh.org).

Getting experience of working in the hospital environment in a role other than a medical practitioner is extremely valuable and can provide valuable insights as well as helping with your career development. In addition, seeing healthcare from different viewpoints may enhance the experiences you gain from your medical course, help you to remember information from your studies and practise communication skills. You will also gain insights into the way other healthcare workers function within the NHS. Not many healthcare assistants have the knowledge of a fourth-year medical student! How about working in a haematology or pathology lab if your interests lie here, or tailoring your healthcare assistant shifts to departments you might like to work in?

Not everybody is aware of the possibility of volunteering, for example over the summer, to help out on a research project in an area of interest to you. This entails speaking to the consultant and nurse specialists in your field of interest, and keeping your eye on the notice boards in that department. Speak to any GPs to whom you are attached as they often have special interests that they are pursuing. Research positions are also advertised on university websites and journals and often pay you for your time.

Shadowing on-call specialist registrars (SpRs) whilst on different rotations and GPs on their out-of-hours shifts is also of great benefit and gives you a much deeper understanding of that specialty.

Although part-time work during term time is often discouraged by medical schools due to the challenging and demanding nature of the course and the amount of study needed, it is often a necessity, and many students have got through the course with a part-time job. The time to quit the job is when you think it may start affecting your work and not when it actually does.

Specialty courses

There are a number of specialty courses which you may have the opportunity to attend that allow you to further your knowledge about specific aspects of medicine. One such course is the Trauma Conference, run by Bart's and the London Queen Mary's School of Medicine every summer. Apart from lectures covering the airway, breathing, circulation (ABC) principles, head injuries, paediatric emergency medicine and conflict medicine, there are extrication demonstrations by the London Fire-brigade Service and practical sessions where students are given the chance to insert intercostal drains and carry out cricothyroidotomies, practise central line insertion and participate in advanced life support (ALS) moulage.[15]

The Royal Society of Medicine also runs over 400 academic meetings, lectures and workshops every year, many of which are free to medical students. There are ample opportunities to further your knowledge in all specialties of medicine as well as if you have a specific field of interest.[16] Student subscription costs around £25 a year.

PasTest runs various courses for medical students as well as doctors at various levels in their career. The company provides over 90 best-selling titles covering all areas of medical revision.[17] For more information *see* Chapter 19.

Many short courses are run by medical schools and royal colleges (*see* Appendix 4); covering a wide variety of subject matter in various specialties throughout the year. For instance, the Royal College of General Practitioners has a series of courses held across the UK on many educational subjects (e.g. skin problems, drug and substance misuse and mental health). Investigate what is available locally, as well as at other universities, as there may be lectures or courses on subjects of interest to you or those you have previously not covered or thought about.

Surgery, medicine and paediatric revision courses are run by the MPS and MDU. These are run on various weekends between January and April every year. Although there are attendance fees, these are discounted if you have signed up with the defence society for your Foundation 1 year.

Finally, to maximise your learning from all these different focused experiences, the *Guidelines for the Delivery of Career Management for Doctors: MMC Working for Career Management*[1] suggests using a range of learning styles to help you reassess and re-evaluate your career choices and progression. You can do this by using:

- reflective logs or journal entries in learning portfolios
- debriefs of experiences in tutorials, with your educational supervisor, through appraisal, or in your peer group
- online focused experience discussions between your peers and senior colleagues
- career handbooks such as this one to help promote your reflection, so do not forget to complete the forms in Appendices 2 and 3 at each of the junctures recommended in Chapter 3.

References

1　Modernising Medical Careers Working Group for Career Management. *Career Management: An Approach for Medical Schools, Deaneries, Royal Colleges and Trusts*. London: Department of Health; 2005.

2　General Medical Council. *Tomorrow's Doctors*. London: GMC; 1993.

3　Ciechan J, Girgis S and Smith P. *The Insiders Guide to Medical School* (7e). Oxford: Blackwell Publishing; 2004.

4　www.keele.ac.uk/depts/ms/undergrad/sscs/index.htm

5　Cross P. Getting the most out of your SSMs. *StudentBMJ*. 2003; **11**: 336–7.

6　Young E, Melvin R, Coombes J et al. Elect to teach. *StudentBMJ*. 2004; **12**: 36.

7　Wilson M. *The Medic's Guide to Work and Electives Around the World* (2e). Oxford: Arnold Publishers; 2004.

8　www.the-mdu.com/ten

9　Bong K. Buddhist medicine in occupied Tibet. *StudentBMJ*. 2004; **12**: 74–5.

10　Clompus H. Grinning in Gambia. *StudentBMJ*. 2004; **12**: 118–19.

11　Rajakumaraswamy N, Toor I and Thomas G. Transferring between medical schools. *StudentBMJ*. 2004; **12**: 20–1.

12　McManus IC, Richards P and Winder BC. Intercalated degrees, learning styles and career preferences: prospective longitudinal study of UK medical students. *BMJ*. 1999; **319**: 542–6.

13　Brown P. Research: what's the point. *StudentBMJ*. 2004; **12**: 46–7.

14　Gray LD. Erasmus: Alpine retreat. *StudentBMJ*. 2003; **11**: 338.

15　www.traumamedicine.org

16　www.rsm.ac.uk/students

17　www.pastest.co.uk

Further reading

www.erasmus.ac.uk/students/studentguide.pdf

www.ifmsa.org

www.ihmec.ucl.ac.uk (elect to teach).

7

Modernising Medical Careers

This chapter introduces the content of the *Modernising Medical Careers* initiative.

What is *Modernising Medical Careers?*[1,2,3,4]

In February 2003, the four UK health departments published a policy statement on *Modernising Medical Careers* (MMC). The aim of the MMC initiative was to improve patient care by delivering a modernised career structure with focused goals and objectives. The structured and streamlined, yet flexible, approach to training was developed to allow trainees to complete training schemes in the shortest time period possible while maintaining their professional competence (Figure 7.1). The structure that the MMC initiative provides ensures that there is less opportunity for 'drifting' to occur within a career.

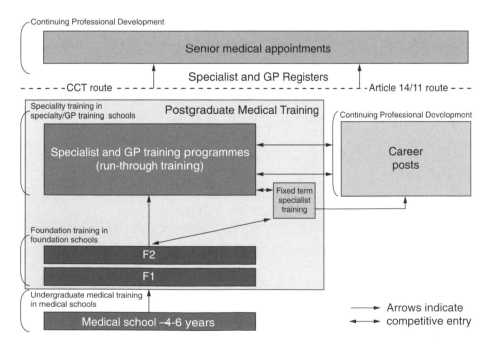

Figure 7.1: UK *Modernising Medical Careers* (MMC) career framework, 2006.

The MMC career framework illustrated in Figure 7.1 outlines the possible career pathways of new medical school graduates and current doctors who are practising in the UK. This may be updated in the future; you will be able to access the most current framework at www.mmc.nhs.uk.

All UK graduates are required to undertake the two-year Foundation Programme (*see below*), and after successful completion of the programme trainees may enter specialist or GP training programmes.

Specialist and GP training programmes are delivered through a range of organisations, supported and overseen by the postgraduate deans. The administrative bodies responsible for delivering the specialist or GP training programmes may be known as a specialty or GP training school. Once doctors enter either of these programmes they have the opportunity to gain a Certificate of Completion of Training (CCT), subject to satisfactory progress. The Postgraduate Medical Education and Training Board (PMETB) has agreed the curricula of the specialist and GP training programmes; it is against the appropriate curriculum that trainees are assessed.

The number of years doctors will spend in training will vary, depending on which programme they have undertaken. Once a doctor has received a CCT they are then legally eligible for entry to the Specialist or GP register and can apply for an appropriate senior medical appointment; this may include GP Principal, other employed GP, consultant or other specialist role.

Doctors who have not completed a specialist or GP training programme may still apply for entry to the Specialist or GP register through the PMETB. Such doctors would have to satisfy the requirements of the PMETB in order to be entered on the appropriate register. This route to the Specialist or GP register may be referred to as the 'Article 14/11 route' (*see* Figure 7.1) because it is defined by articles 11 and 14 of the General and Specialist Medical Practice (Education Training and Qualifications) Order 2003. Once on the register, a doctor applying through this route is then eligible to apply for an appropriate senior medical appointment in the same way as those who are applying via the CCT route.

The MMC initiative ensures quality-assured training. Thus the presence of general competencies, including the ability to manage acutely ill patients, is established using various assessment methods. Doctors training in a Foundation Programme will now have to be able to demonstrate possession of the attitudes and behaviours required to be a good healthcare professional before advancing into a specialist training programme. These competences include accessibility, recognising one's limits, understanding equal opportunities and taking proper responsibility. This focus on competencies also ensures that practitioners can work in all settings, such as primary care and the community, in addition to hospitals. The types of skills which are assessed as a result of the MMC are:

- communication and consultation skills – with patients, families and colleagues
- teamwork – in uni- and multi-professional settings
- establishment and maintenance of effective relationships with patients
- use of evidence and data
- time management
- information technology (IT) skills
- patient safety – this is achieved by ensuring competencies and confidence in skills
- clinical audit.

As a professional training under the new MMC guidance you are more in charge of your own career. The MMC has designed training schemes to be trainee-centred. The advantage of this is that you will know what you are doing each day. To guide you through your training you will have an educational supervisor. The supervisor is not intended to tell you what you should be doing but to help you out if you have any concerns and to provide feedback and advice when necessary.

Another advantage of changes in training, brought about by the MMC, is that you will be able to experience a much wider and specific range of specialties in the Foundation programmes than was previously available in pre-registration house officer (PRHO) posts. Specifically, experience in primary care is available much earlier and more readily than ever before. The aim is for 80% of junior doctor rotations to include general practice by August 2007. This reflects the proportion of health service provision occurring within the community. In addition, areas previously neglected, such as academic medicine and research, will become more accessible. However, because the length of training schemes has been shortened you will have less time to make your career choices. Do not worry that you will be left stranded not knowing what you should be doing to get where you want to be. You should also now be supported by much better career advice throughout your training, as this is an area specifically addressed in the MMC initiative.

What are Foundation Programmes?[5,6]

In 1953, following the Goodenough Report,[5] the PRHO year (the first year as a doctor following graduation from medical school, now known as Foundation Year 1, F1) was introduced as part of medical training to enable application of knowledge and a widening of the new doctor's experience. This was expected to occur with the support of guidance and supervision. In 1975, the PRHO year was criticised by the Merrison Report,[5] which found that it had inadequate organisation, definition of aims and understanding of the proper interaction of the service and education. These issues remained a problem until recently. Part of the reason for this was that the PRHO year had changed very little since its introduction nearly half a century earlier. Therefore the Foundation Programme was designed to address these issues and was launched, in full, for all new doctors who started work in August 2005. To ensure that the Foundation Programme meets adequate standards of training, the curriculum was agreed with the General Medical Council (GMC) and the PMETB.

By placing the onus of completion of objectives on you, the trainee, rather than the trainer, the Foundation Programme has made what was the PRHO year more flexible. However, competency is established in a more structured way through the use of assessments and structured supervision. This type of trainee-led programme equips you with the skills necessary to manage your professional development in the future.

Foundation Year 1 (F1) and Foundation Year 2 (F2) make up the two-year Foundation Programme which all UK medical graduates are required to undertake before progressing to specialty or GP training. The Foundation Programme usually consists of six, four-month attachments. It is the first of these two years (F1) that is equivalent to the old-style PRHO year. During F1 you are required to have a rotation in surgery and in medicine. You will also have protected, 'bleep-free' time for planned learning. F2 is equivalent to the first year of the old-style senior house officer (SHO) post, in which you can build upon the skills and knowledge you acquired in F1. As with the pre-Foundation training, you will receive provisional registration from the GMC upon graduation and you will qualify for full GMC registration after successful completion of the F1 year. Although true at the time of printing, this may change, as the GMC is in consultation about an outcome-based programme for which successful completion would be required before full registration may take place. If this were to go ahead, provisional registration would occur at the same time but full registration may occur anywhere between graduation and completion of Foundation training. The current situation is that all medical graduates are required to complete the Foundation Programme in order to work as a doctor in the UK.

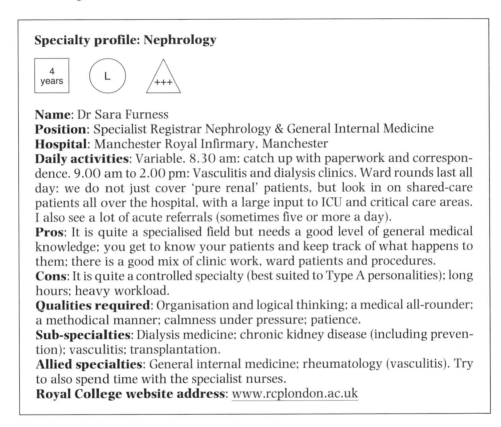

Specialty profile: Nephrology

Name: Dr Sara Furness
Position: Specialist Registrar Nephrology & General Internal Medicine
Hospital: Manchester Royal Infirmary, Manchester
Daily activities: Variable. 8.30 am: catch up with paperwork and correspondence. 9.00 am to 2.00 pm: Vasculitis and dialysis clinics. Ward rounds last all day: we do not just cover 'pure renal' patients, but look in on shared-care patients all over the hospital, with a large input to ICU and critical care areas. I also see a lot of acute referrals (sometimes five or more a day).
Pros: It is quite a specialised field but needs a good level of general medical knowledge; you get to know your patients and keep track of what happens to them; there is a good mix of clinic work, ward patients and procedures.
Cons: It is quite a controlled specialty (best suited to Type A personalities); long hours; heavy workload.
Qualities required: Organisation and logical thinking; a medical all-rounder; a methodical manner; calmness under pressure; patience.
Sub-specialties: Dialysis medicine; chronic kidney disease (including prevention); vasculitis; transplantation.
Allied specialties: General internal medicine; rheumatology (vasculitis). Try to also spend time with the specialist nurses.
Royal College website address: www.rcplondon.ac.uk

So, what are the general expectations of you in your F1 year? Although it is a bridge to your future, the following are expected of you during your F1 year:

- you should be able to put your knowledge, skills and attitudes, learnt at medical school, into practice
- you should be gaining new knowledge and skills; a particular focus of the Foundation Programme is acquisition of the skills required to recognise and manage acutely ill patients
- you should be fine-tuning your professional attitudes.

Completion of the Foundation Programme requires you to demonstrate progress in the standards set out by the GMC in a document called *The New Doctor* (*see* Chapter 9). Assessments used are described in full at www.mmc.nhs.uk; however, they include the following.

- Multi-source feedback (there are two tools in use, dependent on the deanery at which you are training):
  - mini-peer assessment tool (mini-PAT) – you will have to nominate eight assessors from your team, nursing staff or allied health professional colleagues

    to fill out a questionnaire that is returned anonymously; you will also have to complete a self-assessment using the same questionnaire

- team assessment of behaviour (TAB) – you will have to select ten co-workers to assess you using 360° TAB forms with envelopes addressed to the Foundation Training Programme Director (FTPD) to enable anonymous return of the form; your assessors should include at least five qualified nurses, preferably ward sister level, and three doctors, including the current supervising consultant or GP.

• Direct observation of doctor–patient interaction:
- mini-clinical evaluation exercise (mini-CEX) – a 15-minute observed encounter with a patient in order to assess your clinical skills, attitudes, behaviours and ability to provide good patient care
- direct observation of procedural skills (DOPS) – a structured checklist to assess your practical skills.

• Case-based discussion (CBD) – a structured discussion with your supervisor about a clinical case you are involved in to establish your clinical reasoning and judgement skills.

Following successful completion of F2, you will receive a Foundation Achievement of Competency Document (FACD), which you will require in order to start higher training positions.

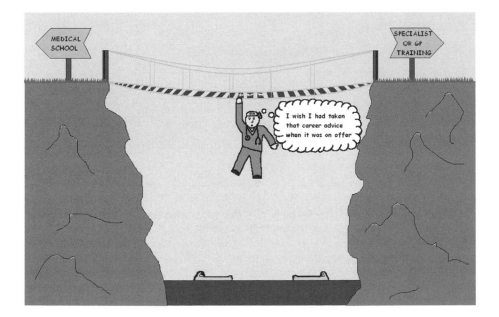

Postgraduate deaneries and Foundation schools

The UK has been divided up geographically into 'deaneries'. A postgraduate dean heads each deanery. Each deanery has responsibility for the delivery of the Foundation Programme training in its area, through Foundation schools. A Foundation School is not the same as a postgraduate medical school. It does not represent a building but a number of institutions, grouped together to offer the required variety of placements to ensure complete and wide education and training. Within a Foundation School there will be acute and mental health trusts, general practices, universities and other relevant institutions, such as hospices and public health departments (*see* Figure 7.2).

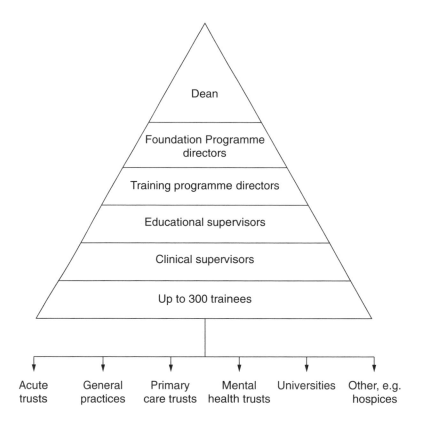

Figure 7.2:   The structure of Foundation schools.

Specifically, each deanery must ensure that the standards set by the GMC and the PMETB are being met. The deaneries in the UK are:

- Eastern
- Kent, Sussex and Surrey
- Leicester, Northamptonshire and Rutland (LNR)
- London
- Mersey
- Northern

- Northern Ireland
- Northwestern
- Oxford
- Scotland (divided into East, West, North and South-east regions)
- Severn and Wessex
- South Yorkshire and Humberside
- Peninsula
- Trent
- Yorkshire
- Wales
- West Midlands.

Some of the deaneries may merge together in 2006/2007 as a consequence of the restructuring of the NHS in England. Therefore you should obtain up-to-date information from the COPMED website (www.copmed.org.uk/contacts/).

It is important that you familiarise yourself with the roles of a postgraduate deanery, which include:

- provision of information about and recruitment to the Foundation Programme
- arranging shadowing and/or induction periods prior to starting F1 (*see* Chapter 10 for more information on shadowing periods)
- establishing that local assessment procedures are in accordance with national procedures
- ensuring that regular and appropriate appraisals occur
- ensuring that those undertaking assessments receive adequate training
- provision of appropriate career management and development opportunities and advice to enable a smooth progression of trainees from F1 to F2.

Specialty profile: Neurology

| 5 years | L | ⚠ ++ |

Name: Dr Anthony Kenton
Position: Consultant Neurologist
Hospital: University Hospitals Coventry and Warwickshire (Walsgrave Hospital), Warwick
Daily activities: Per week I do three outpatient clinics; 2–3 ward rounds; 3–4 academic or business meetings; teaching students and administration. But there is no such thing as a typical day!
Qualities required: None are essential! But you must be able to cope with not having quick fixes!
Pros: Interesting diseases; long term management of patients (e.g. epilepsy, Parkinson's); few inpatients so lots of time to discuss cases; on-call is non-resident as a registrar; smallish department so some autonomy; good prospects for teaching students or junior doctors, etc.
Cons: Lots of non-organic disease (dizzy spells, tension headache, etc.); not enough junior grades to run a proper on-call service; lots of pressure on clinic waiting times.

Sub-specialties: Stroke neurology (as I do); multiple sclerosis; movement disorders; epilepsy; nerve/muscle disease; headache; neurorehabilitation.
Allied specialties: Neurophysiology; neurosurgery; neurorehabilitation; psychiatry.
Royal College website address: www.rcplondon.ac.uk

Inter-deanery transfer

Inter-deanery transfer describes the process by which you may change your postgraduate deanery from the one that originally accepted you. Often, this will occur at the beginning of F1 or F2. Otherwise you are automatically expected to work in the deanery that covers the area of your medical school.

Inter-deanery transfer is not a situation that should occur without good reason. In order for you to undertake an inter-deanery transfer, there must be available posts in the receiving deanery and you must be able to satisfy your original and your new deaneries that your reason for changing is good. 'Well-founded' reasons, deemed as acceptable circumstances in which inter-deanery transfers may occur, include:

- health reasons
- carer responsibilities
- in order to pursue research opportunities.

Inter-deanery transfers may not be so much of an issue now that the medical training application service (MTAS) has been introduced. All applicants are asked to rank all 27 UK Foundation Schools in their application, thus resulting in the possibility of being placed at any.

Application and selection process

One of the aims of the *Modernising Medical Careers* initiative was to simplify, standardise and co-ordinate recruitment and selection for the Foundation Programmes and further specialist or GP posts. As a result, the selection process used for recruitment of Foundation doctors has been designed to be open, fair and legally robust. Educationalists and recruitment specialists have designed the application and selection processes, thus ensuring these goals are met.

Application to the Foundation Programme involves standardised documentation, such as application forms, to ensure the process is fair for all applicants. The word 'transparent' is often used to describe the application process; this means that it is easy to demonstrate how a decision will be/has been reached. There are clear instructions for completion of the application forms and marking criteria are available to all applicants.

The application and selection processes for Foundation Programmes and specialist/GP posts have been brought into line to allow successful 'Foundation doctors' to be able to directly enter specialist or GP posts. Recruitment has been co-ordinated nationally to allow smooth progression through training for all doctors, even if they want to move around within the country.

Further information on the application and selection processes for Foundation Programmes (and beyond) can be found at www.mtas.nhs.uk and www. mmc.nhs.uk.

References

1 Modernising Medical Careers. *Rough Guide: Foundation years*, 2005. (Available from www.mmc.nhs.uk/download_files/The-Rough-Guide-to-the-Foundation-Programme.pdf)

2 MacDonald R. Modernising Medical Careers. *StudentBMJ*. 2003; **11**: 372–3.

3 Department of Health. *Modernising Medical Careers: the next steps*. London: Department of Health; 2004.

4 Modernising Medical Careers. *New Training Programme Heralds a New Era in UK Medicine*, 2005. (Available from www.mmc.nhs.uk/pages/news/article?D2E8271F-1C0D-4199-A980-B84D46B716C8)

5 General Medical Council. *The New Doctor: recommendations on general clinical training*, 2005. (Available from www.gmc-uk.org/education/foundation/new_doctor.asp)

6 Modernising Medical Careers. *Frequently Asked Questions*. (Available from www.mmc.nhs.uk/pages/foundation/FAQ)

Further reading

British Medical Association. *Guidance on Applying for Foundation Programmes*. London: BMA; 2005.

Conference of Postgraduate Medical Deans of the United Kingdom (www.copmed.org.uk). (Includes among other things links to many career-related and institution websites)

8

Foundation Programme pilots

The concept of the Foundation Programme for junior doctors is relatively new. Deaneries have, therefore, piloted Foundation programmes in advance of them 'going live' in 2005–2006. The first cohort entered Foundation Year 1 (F1) in August 2005. They will move into Foundation Year 2 in August 2006. Deaneries have been evaluating their pilot programmes and collecting data (such as on the quality of training placements, the education programmes and assessment tools). They have been learning about successes and problems. This chapter highlights the findings from the Foundation Programme pilots in an attempt to provide you with information, reassurance and the answers to some concerns you may have.

Many medical students facing the prospect of starting their career under the relatively new Foundation Programme initiative may be apprehensive. You may have heard rumours both positive and negative. So how can you prepare yourself for what is inevitably ahead? Data currently available to answer this question were produced following pilots of Foundation programmes.

Between 2003 and 2005, pilots of the Foundation Programme were organised within deaneries across England. As a result, 11 reports were produced, covering to varying degrees, placement length, induction, supervision, specialty choices, tasters, teaching, general practice exposure, assessment and portfolio and career management. These reports were summarised in a review that provides the basis of this chapter.[1]

Three reports considered Foundation Year 1 (F1) and Foundation Year 2 (F2): one report considered F1 alone and seven considered the F2 period alone.[1] The results of these reports have been summarised in Table 8.1. This table details the worries and findings of the pilot study results, to give you an impression of the problems you may still face and to reassure you. It tells you what lies ahead and allows you to be more alert to problems with the programme early on, when you can still do something about them.

Table 8.1: Summary of Foundation Programme pilot findings[1]

	Worries or problems identified	General findings
Four-month placement length	Difficulty integrating with teams (unfounded)	Four-month placements did not produce problems with integration
	Less attractive to trainees who have a clear idea of their future career	F1 trainees generally more unhappy with placement length than F2 trainees
		Shorter placements provided wider experience, more information on career options and a holistic view
Nature of placements	Duplication of activities and experiences of F1 or F2 (unfounded)	A&E and acute medicine were useful for core and clinical skills
	Specialised or busy placements were sometimes unsuccessful	'Tasters' (up to two weeks in one specialty) were excellent
	Trainees sometimes viewed as students rather than doctors in GP placements	F2 placements were most successful for trainees uncertain about their future career direction
Induction period	Need to be creative, rather than just being 'talked at'	Short, two-day induction worked well
	Clearer guidance/information requested	
Educational supervisors and supervision	Time a major issue preventing adequate work with trainees	Trainee doctors valued supervision
	Not all consultants who were involved in supervision understood the *Modernising Medical Careers* initiative and Foundation training	Trainee doctors felt they learnt more as a result of supervision
	Quality of supervision may have been reduced as a result of inadequate training	Supervision was generally better in community and GP placements
Taught components	Attendance was a major problem in nearly all deaneries	Interactive 'hands-on' sessions were more popular
	Topics such as ethics and professional behaviour duplicated areas covered at medical school	Multi-professional teaching was well-received in most deaneries
Assessment and administration	Assessments resulted in problematic extra work for clinical and educational supervisors	360° (multi-source) feedback was a positive experience for trainees and their colleagues
	Administration required an additional employee to avoid delays	

Table 8.1: Continued

	Worries or problems identified	General findings
	Some trainees found it difficult to get their competencies signed off Assessments were sometimes viewed as over the top without a clear educational purpose	
Career management	Nearly all deaneries recognised this as an area requiring development	The proportion of trainees undecided about their future career wishes reduced after the Foundation pilot
	More structure and specificity was needed	Placements and attachments supported career choice
GP placements for all	Educational support and space was identified as a problem	Provided useful career information Increased the number of trainees placing general practice as their no.1 career choice (in *most* deaneries)
Portfolio	Time-consuming	Use of a workbook or portfolio was found by many deaneries to be invaluable
	Too much paperwork	Precise and concise documentation is essential
	Unclear as to best use for it (since this finding a new portfolio has been created and this has been well-received)	
Service impact	Worries about a negative impact on service because of absence for teaching sessions, supervision and assessments	Holistic approach to patient care
		More information may be found at www.mmc.nhs.uk/pages/foundation/pilot-results

Reference

1 National Health Service. *Pilot Evaluation Review: a review of the pilot evaluations in England conducted from the end of 2002 through to 2005.* London: Modernising Medical Careers; 2005.

9

Application to Foundation Year posts

Despite reassurance that the ratio of Foundation jobs to medical school graduates favours successful application to junior doctor jobs, this situation appears set to change. In addition, the number of jobs nationwide is irrelevant if you want to undertake your Foundation training in a specific area. There is an excess of Foundation programmes over the number of doctors graduating from UK medical schools. The number of Foundation programmes is increasing year on year to accommodate the increasing number of graduates. But, because of European law, there is a potential problem because of the potential influx of European graduates applying for Foundation programmes in the UK. Some areas also produce more medical students than there are Foundation programmes in their localities, for example London and Leicester, which means that not all their students will be able to stay local to where they went to medical school. Competition for Foundation Programme places in these areas for students from outside medical schools will be fierce. Conversely, other areas, such as the West Midlands, have to actively attract students into their region for Foundation training. This chapter aims to help you with your Foundation application, from choosing rotations best-suited to you to giving you guidance as to what you should be doing and when.

So, the time has come. You are facing the daunting prospect of applying for your first job as a doctor. First, some good news, in 2005 the UK had around 10% 'headroom', that is 10% more Foundation Year 1 (F1) posts than the output from medical schools;[1] even better, the British Medical Association (BMA) was quoting this figure as being around 12% in 2006. However, that is where the good news may be set to change. Headroom is dynamic, and with medical schools continuing to over-recruit, the BMA is concerned that previous 'headroom' figures look set to nearly halve in 2007, with further reductions in subsequent years.

The Foundation Programme is relatively new. Therefore, changes to the programme itself and to the application procedure may occur. The information provided in this chapter is based on the recruitment process of Foundation Year 1 (F1) trainees starting in August 2006. You will have to refer to the MMC website (www.mmc.nhs.uk) for the most up to date information.

How to choose deaneries and rotations that will suit you

The first step in the application process is to apply to a Foundation School – you have to rank all 27 UK Foundation Schools in the order of your preference. Once accepted at a Foundation School (and armed with your application score) you have to rank the rotations on offer into your preferred order. Where do you start? There are a number of ways in which you can answer this question, depending on your priorities. Think about what is important to you and what you want to get from the job. Below are a number of factors that you may want to consider now and in the future when you are choosing more senior posts:

- Location of training (important for choosing your Foundation School):
  - Geographical area – do you have family commitments or dependents? Do you want to change to somewhere new or stick to where you know? Certain areas in the country have more competion for jobs than others. Information on this can be gained by referring to www.bmjcareers.com/cgi-bin/section.pl?sn=juniorcomp.
- Type of hospital and thus experience[3] (important when choosing rotations):
  - District general hospital – may provide more experience as you will be busy and the 'patient mix' is general and representative of the normal distribution of disorders. The senior staff to junior staff ratio is generally lower.
- Specialty interest – although you do not need to decide exactly what you want to do right now, you may want more experience in your specialty of interest or its allied specialties (*see* relevant specialty profiles throughout the text). If you have completed the form 'Current career interests', in Appendix 2, it would be useful to refer to it at this stage. Do not worry if you do not lean towards any particular subject, as Foundation years are designed to give you a wide breadth of experience to later build on and specialise further.
- Opportunity for job satisfaction and career progression.
- Work–life balance – you can try and speak to junior doctors already in the jobs you are considering. In addition, read the flexible training section in Chapter 12.
- Money – for more information on this consult Chapter 12. Although details of banding and exact salaries are not readily available from deaneries at the application stage, you may be able to talk to current employees.
- Publishing potential – specialties such as public health often provide good opportunities for getting work published. Some consultants have a notable interest in research. You can enquire about this at the hospital or check on the relevant hospital's website.
- Confidence – it is not a good idea to rule out posts because you are not confident in the skills required. These can be practised and you will gain a lot from a rotation you are weaker in. However, it is important you are realistic! Identify any relevant weaknesses you may have so you can address them, and practise specific skills, before you start in the position if you can.

Once you have considered the above, and any other personal priorities, you should research where appropriate. Try visiting the hospital, talking to staff and exploring the local area. Attempt to visualise yourself within each post, including the travelling, the nature of the work and colleagues with whom you would be working. This may help you to focus on aspects of the job not covered above. After this take another look at the rotations on offer and see if your decision is clearer. If all this fails Houghton[4] suggests taking notice of your gut reaction when choosing jobs!

Application advice

Once the application process is open, you are asked to indicate your preferred Foundation School by placing this first in your ranking of all 27 in the UK. Each Foundation School is applied to using a standardised and structured application form, available on-line. Your university will organise a statement of eligibility and academic record/cause for concern; however, it is your responsibility to chase this up. Initially, for the majority of Foundation Schools you will usually only be applying to F1 jobs. Foundation year 2 (F2) job applications generally occur 6-9 months into the F1 year.[2] Despite the timing of the F2 applications, the good news is that all successful F1 trainees are currently *guaranteed* an F2 post within the same Foundation School.

In addition to personal and demographic information you will need to provide two referees. It is important that these referees are people with whom you have worked recently and closely, preferably senior medical tutors. They will be emailed a pro-forma to complete to validate your application. Thus, it is essential that they can honestly confirm your clinical abilities.

The main part of your application comprises a personal statement consisting of a number of headings. You should submit relevant comments under each heading which must adhere to a strict word count. Each heading is scored individually. You must support your comments with evidence that demonstrates your knowledge, understanding and experience in a number of specified areas relating to the General Medical Council's (GMC) document *Good Medical Practice*:[6] academic achievements, non-academic achievements, *The New Doctor* guidelines,[7] personal and education reasons for applying to first ranked Foundation School/deanery or programme, teamwork and leadership. Check carefully that there are no spelling mistakes and computer errors – they do not look professional! Detailed information about individual questions on the form can be found through www.mmc.nhs.uk. Keep a copy of the form you send in, as this information may be used later, for example in an interview (if applicable).

Panels, associated with the Foundation School you have applied to, will score your statements. This is done anonymously, and results in one final score that takes you through the application process. If your score does not result in a job offer from your first choice Foundation School, your documentation will be passed on to your second-ranked Foundation School and so forth until all available places have been allocated.

The Medical Training Application Service (MTAS) has a single deadline for submitting the application, which is usually in November. The following two points are crucial:

- Honesty is essential when applying for your Foundation jobs. A random audit of all applications is undertaken. If you make false claims you will be reported to the GMC and your career may be over before it has even started.

- If you are offered a programme you are obliged to accept this. Otherwise you can be reported to the GMC, which would jeopardise your career.

Devolved nations

The application process outlined above applies mainly to England. If you want to apply to Scotland, Northern Ireland or Wales and do not already live there, the following information may be useful. However, you will still need a letter of support from your university and/or postgraduate deanery as this is a GMC requirement.

Scotland

In Scotland you apply using the Scottish Foundation Allocation Scheme (SFAS), which works as a two-phase online matching scheme much like MDAP. Deadlines for applications to Foundation programmes may be different between Scotland and the rest of the UK.

You can rank up to four Foundation programmes, and will need to submit a number of additional forms, including separate ones for registration, application, equal opportunities, applicant ranking, and a CV. More information and the forms can be found on the SFAS website (www.nes.scot.nhs.uk/sfas).

Specialty profile: Obstetrics and gynaecology

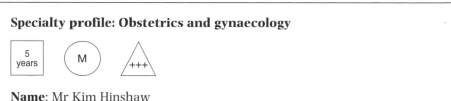

Name: Mr Kim Hinshaw
Position: Consultant Obstetrician and Gynaecologist
Hospital: Sunderland Royal Hospital, Tyne and Wear
Daily activities: My normal clinical work is done from 9 am till 5 pm Monday to Thursday. The week is varied and includes one major operating list, one alternate weekday case list, one gynaecology outpatient clinic, two ante-natal clinics (including one looking after 'high-risk' obstetric cases), one labour ward session and one obstetric ultrasound clinic (including invasive procedures – amniocentesis, etc.). My interests in undergraduate teaching, research and postgraduate education take up the rest of my week. I have a private gynae-cology clinic for a couple of hours after work on a Tuesday – this does not eat into family time too much and pays for the 'extras'!
Qualities required: Enthusiasm, good communication skills and effective teamworking are essential as we work with many other disciplines and professionals.

Pros: Day-to-day clinical work is varied; large centres see plenty of interesting clinical cases; supportive department; you are encouraged to develop special interest areas; undergraduate and postgraduate teaching opportunities. The trust is very supportive of my interests outside the immediate clinical area (Chair of the Regional Postgraduate Training Committee and national/international lecturing).

Cons: Frustrations with meeting arbitrary targets that clinicians do not always feel are 'patient friendly'; finding time to fit in clinical work, administration, teaching, lecturing, training, research, family, friends and outside interests! Part of the problem is curtailing my own enthusiasm and making sure my work–life balance is right.

Sub-specialties: Presently, core competencies in both obstetrics and gynaecology are required to become a consultant; eventually consultants orientate to one or the other and develop special interests; in larger hospitals there is often a formal split. *Obstetrics*: 'high-risk' pregnancy; labour ward management; feto-maternal medicine (including obstetric ultrasound) and maternal medicine. *Gynaecology*: minimally invasive surgery (laparoscopic and hysteroscopic); infertility; pelvic floor or uro-gynaecology; gynaecological oncology (including colposcopy); gynaecological endocrine/menopause; sexual and reproductive health. *Academic*: research or teaching is a major component of the job. *The future*: whether the specialty will totally split is not yet clear. Major changes in gynaecological practice in the last 10 years mean fewer hysterectomies are done for menstrual problems. Generalist consultants of the near future will mainly be an obstetrician and 'office' gynaecologist (will offer emergency gynaecology cover but will only undertake minor and intermediate elective surgery).

Allied specialties: Neonatology/paediatrics; primary care; general medicine; anaesthetics (ITU); general surgery. Electives spent in developing countries are often very productive in terms of hands-on experience in acute obstetrics. It is no longer necessary to undertake formal training outside the specialty in order to become a consultant.

Royal College website address: www.rcog.org.uk

Wales and Northern Ireland

In Wales and Northern Ireland (NI) there is a single point of entry to their national allocation schemes. In NI you rank and apply to three hospitals that will offer two-year training. In Wales you apply to the All Wales Foundation School and can be allocated posts anywhere in Wales.

Timeline for Foundation Programme application events

Figure 9.1 is intended as a rough guide to the timeline of events occurring as part of your Foundation Programme application. You will have to consult www.mmc.nhs.uk for accurate and up-to-date information.

Summary of GMC guidelines

This section of this *Handbook* may trigger a groan, and that is just from those of you who have continued to read this far! However, despite the idea of reading guidelines as being time-consuming, dry and boring, it is vitally important that all medical students and healthcare professionals are aware of the content of the various GMC guidelines.

You are accountable to the GMC, and straying from the medical practice outlined in its guidelines will risk your professional registration and ultimately may result in you losing your job. Even as a medical student you are expected to behave and act in accordance with GMC guidance. Below are the edited highlights of the titled guidelines; by no means does this substitute reading the guidance provided by the GMC. This section serves as an introduction and, after you have read the full guidance, it will be a source of reference to jog your memory of the content of each.

Duties of a doctor

This is fairly self-explanatory. The GMC states that the required qualities of all doctors are to:[6]

*   make the *care* of your patient your first concern
*   treat every patient *politely* and *considerately*
*   respect patients' *dignity* and *privacy*
*   *listen* to patients and respect their views
*   give patients *information* in a way they can understand
*   *respect* the rights of patients to be fully involved in decisions about their care
*   keep your professional *knowledge* and *skills* up to date
*   be *honest* and *trustworthy*
*   respect and *protect confidential information*
*   make sure that your personal beliefs do *not prejudice* your patients' care
*   act quickly to *protect patients from risk* if you have good reason to believe that you or a colleague may not be fit to practise

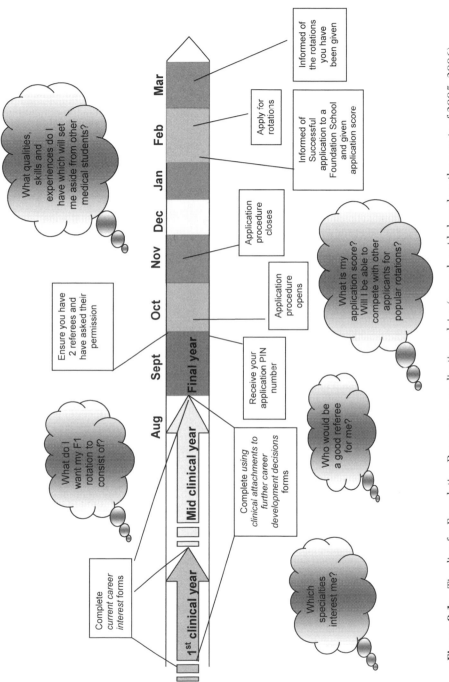

Figure 9.1: Timeline for Foundation Programme application advice (a rough guide based on the events of 2005–2006).

- *avoid abusing your position* as a doctor
- *work with colleagues* in ways that best serve patients' interests
- *never discriminate unfairly* against patients or colleagues
- always be prepared to *justify your actions.*

Good Medical Practice

The *Good Medical Practice* booklet,[6] initially published in 1995 and revised in 2001, is an indexed document which expands on the duties of a doctor. It sets out guidelines, principles and standards of competent, professional care and conduct, under seven main headings. The headings are as follows.

Good clinical care

You must:

- practise good standards of clinical care – this includes assessing, investigating and treating patients adequately and when necessary
- practise within the limits of your ability – you must be able to recognise your own limits and competencies
- make sure patients are not put at unnecessary risks – only provide treatment when adequate knowledge of the patient's health or medical needs has been obtained.

Maintaining good medical practice

You must:

- stay up-to-date with developments in your field – including knowledge of laws and statutory codes of practice
- maintain your skills
- ensure cover is arranged when you are off duty
- ensure you have adequate insurance or professional indemnity cover (*see* Chapter 19).

Relationships with patients

You must:

- be able to develop, encourage and maintain trust, confidentiality, communication and successful relationships with your patients.

Working with colleagues

You must:

- work effectively with colleagues in medicine, other healthcare professionals and allied healthcare workers – treat them with respect and share appropriate information
- ensure you take up posts you have formally accepted
- know how to delegate and refer patient care.

Teaching and training

You:

- have teaching responsibilities to colleagues, patients and their relatives – you should be willing to contribute to the education of students and colleagues
- must develop the skills, attitudes and practices of a competent teacher.

Probity

You must:

- be honest – including at times of mistakes or misadventure.

Health

You must:

- maintain your health
- take appropriate steps to make sure your own health does not put patients, colleagues or the public at risk.

Please note that at the time of writing the GMC is reviewing its *Good Medical Practice* guidelines and the revised edition should be published late in 2006.

The New Doctor

The current guidance, entitled *The New Doctor*,[5] is effective from January 2005 until July 2007. The guidelines describe the seven standards, outlined in *Good Medical Practice*,[7] which should be followed in your first year after graduation, your F1 year.
   Areas covered within this guidance include the following.

- Curriculum content, structure and delivery:
    - identifies clear learning outcomes for training
    - provides information on assessing junior doctors' performance and competence: competencies that are required before full registration can be granted are listed and explained; makes strict assessment of F1 doctors necessary before they are allowed to gain full registration
    - covers areas concerning health and conduct.
- Frameworks to:
    - design training programmes
    - assess F1 doctors
    - recruit F1 doctors.
- Responsibilities of different organisations.

References

1 Malawana J. Laying good foundations. *StudentBMJ*. 2005; **12**: 328–9.

2 *Modernising Medical Careers. Frequently Asked Questions*. (Available from www.mmc.nhs.uk/faq.asp?sector=faq)

3 Westall J. Choosing a house job. *BMJ Career Focus*. 1999; **318**: 2.

4 Houghton A. Getting that job: deciding to apply. *StudentBMJ*. 2003; **11**: 376.

5 General Medical Council. *The New Doctor: recommendations on general clinical training*, 2005. (Available from www.gmc-uk.org/med_ed/newdoc.htm)

6 General Medical Council. *Good Medical Practice*, 2001. (Available from www.gmc-uk.org/med-ed/default.htm)

7 General Medical Council. *The Duties of a Doctor Registered with the General Medical Council*. (Available from www.gmc-uk.org/standards/doad.htm)

Further reading

British Medical Association. *Guidance on Applying for Foundation Programmes*. London: BMA; 2005.

Thomson J. Pre-registration house jobs in general practice. *BMJ Career Focus*. 1998; **317**: 2. (Good article for information on GP junior doctor jobs)

Medical Students Committee. Final report: BMA final year member views on application to Foundation Programmes. London, British Medical Association; 2006.

10

The consolidation period

This chapter will provide you with an overview of what the consolidation period is and what happens during this time.

Although a 'consolidation period' may manifest itself in different ways in different medical schools, and be called a variety of names, this chapter uses the term in a generic way. The consolidation period relates to a time, usually near the end of your course, during which the main aims are to:

- round off undergraduate learning to ensure students are ready for their final exams
- facilitate the transition from medical student to junior doctor
- prepare for a lifetime of continuing learning.

Specialty profile: Oncology

| 4 years | M | +++ |

Name: Dr Jane Worlding
Position: Consultant Clinical Oncologist
Hospital: University Hospitals of Coventry & Warwick, Warwickshire
Daily activities: Clinic work most days: new patient clinic, outpatients, chemotherapy clinic, radiotherapy planning and review clinic; weekly ward round; administration.
Qualities required: Good communication skills; patience; empathy; being able to work in a team; an interest in CT, MRI and technical aspects of radiotherapy planning.
Pros: Varied from day to day; good continuity of care for individual patients; technically challenging; technology and computer use involved in radio-therapy planning is enjoyable.
Cons: Can be draining as many patients die eventually.
Sub-specialties: For example urological, colorectal and skin malignancies; carcinoid tumours.
Allied specialties: Either surgical or physician training complement oncology; radiology would also be useful.
Royal College website address: www.rcplondon.ac.uk

The beginning of the consolidation period may be spent revising for, then sitting, your final exams. Your tutors at your university hospital(s) may provide revision sessions. However, the most help will be gained from continuing to practise clinical skills.

Below, two junior doctors discuss their shadowing experience in this consolidation period.

Name: Dr Kathleen Mackie

Age: 21+ years
Position: Foundation Year 1 (F1) doctor
Hospital: University Hospital of North Staffordshire
Specialty in which shadowing took place: Vascular surgery.
What shadowing involved: Basically, doing the job of a F1 doctor, i.e. clerking in patients, doing simple procedures, etc.
A typical day: My experience of shadowing the F1 doctor was great. I (initially) thought four weeks was too long, especially as I had just finished my finals and wanted to start my summer holiday, but the time flew by. A typical day involved learning how my consultant likes to do things. I learnt what antibiotic regimens they liked, their anticoagulation preferences and other such useful information that made starting my job much easier. I also had to decide the order of the operating list for the next day. Other information that you learn each day whilst shadowing is which tests to order, how to get them done and how to act on their results. During the shadowing block I also met other medical students who were about to start their jobs in the same hospital. This meant that on our first day there were fewer faces that we had never seen before. As a result of completing my shadowing period I did not feel as lost or isolated as I could have done when I started my first post.
Advice for students: Good luck to you all, and enjoy your shadowing period.

Name: Dr Milan M Mehta

Age: 24 years
Position: Medical Senior House Officer
Hospital and specialty in which shadowing occurred: Royal Bolton Hospital (PRHO Medicine, on gastroenterology ward).
What shadowing involved: Thinking what would I do when I had to fill the shoes of the then house officer a few weeks later, for example skills I had to learn or practise.
A typical day: 8.45 am – Help the PRHO chase up the latest blood results and mentally prepare ourselves for the consultant ward round to start shortly; 9 am – consultant ward round. I presented some of the patients that I clerked the day before. Whilst the PRHO presented the rest of the patients, I listed the ward round jobs; 10.30 am – the PRHO and I split the ward round jobs. I did any venflons and important blood tests that needed doing. He let me do the 'exciting' procedures (e.g. an ascitic/pleural tap or a femoral stab). I also got practice at re-writing drug charts and doing lots of discharge letters; 12 noon – lunch; 2 pm

– second consultant ward round and, again, split the ward round jobs with the PRHO; 3.30 pm – I went home early.

Advice for students: (1) Each day ask the ward sister to tell you about the sickest patients, any new patients and then the rest of the patients, and your job will be to see the patients in that order of priority; (2) Always stay on the right side of the nurses as they have a lot of experience and will guide you through your first few weeks as a PRHO, and will often go out of their way to help you out; (3) Probably the single most important skill you need to learn as a PRHO is how to manage your time effectively.

An important aim of the final year is to facilitate the transition from being a medical student to working as a junior doctor. In the consolidation period most students have the opportunity to shadow the house officer whom they will succeed in the following August. The length of this period will vary between medical schools; however, it often ranges from one week to one month. This period is included in the number of weeks of clinical training required by the GMC for provisional registration. Therefore, attendance is compulsory. Shadowing will assist students to acquire a working knowledge of their first post before taking over full responsibility for it.

At the beginning of the shadowing period most students should meet their Foundation year educational supervisor, in addition to the house officer from whom they will be taking over. This contact with your future educational supervisor is designed to continue throughout the first post. Such early contact will provide support and allow you, as a medical student, to establish a pattern for your continuing supervision.

11

What's good about a career in medicine?

Life as a doctor can be difficult. Colleagues, peers and other professionals moan about their work, life, pay and patients. The aim of this chapter is to provide you with the reasons why it is worth continuing in the medical profession and the benefits of working in the NHS.

To realise why it is a great time to be working in the National Health Service (NHS) you should first consider the main criticisms of working in the NHS and why they are becoming less valid.

Most doctors who have left the NHS blamed the poor lifestyle and low pay as their main reasons for leaving. However, Chapter 12 illustrates how these complaints are being vigorously tackled. Junior doctors' pay is now protected by the 'New Deal',[1] which results in them being paid for the hours that they work. The more antisocial hours you work the greater the supplement to your pay. You could end up being paid an extra 80% of your basic wage. The introduction of the European Working Time Directive (EWTD)[2] has resulted in junior doctors' hours being protected. In simple terms, they can no longer be made to work exhaustingly long hours. In fact, by 2009 the maximum hours a junior doctor will be allowed to work per week will be 48, a lot less than the 90+ hours per week of old! With the introduction of flexible working you can work part-time without the fear of losing out on training.

The NHS doctors' representative organisations and doctors themselves realise that doctors need lives outside medicine. They need time with their families and to maintain other pursuits. The aim of the 'Improving Working Lives' initiative[3] is to let doctors live balanced lives. It sets out a standard against which staff can measure their trust's management of human resources. NHS organisations must prove how they are trying to improve the working lives of their employees.

No one can guarantee that by becoming a doctor you will have a brilliant life. However, what you can be sure of is that you will work in an environment that thrives on teamwork and close relationships. You will be immersed in a culture that believes in working and playing hard. However, there will always be people there to support for you if your work or play begins to affect your life negatively, for example the Royal Medical Benevolent Fund (RMBF).[4]

Specialty profile: Orthopaedics

6 years	H	∆ +++

Name: Mr Mohamed Arafa

Position: Consultant Orthopaedic Surgeon; Honorary Clinical Senior Lecturer; Associate Postgraduate Dean

Hospital: The Alexandra Hospital, Redditch (clinical work); Birmingham University (undergraduate); West Midlands Deanery, Birmingham (postgraduate)

Daily activities: I am an early bird! I usually start my pre-operative or post-operative ward round at 7.45 am. I see my secretary to sign letters, respond to correspondence and so on, before going to the theatre or outpatients clinic at 9 am. I may have a meeting or a lecture at lunchtime. In the afternoon, I am either in theatre, outpatient clinic or at my office at the West Midlands Deanery. Very important aspects of my daily work are bedside teaching on ward rounds, in outpatient clinics and hands-on training in the operating theatre of the junior doctors. I run my private practice in the evening and the weekend. I spend one to two hours every evening browsing the internet for teaching materials, responding to e-mails and preparing lectures, etc.

Qualities required: Manual dexterity; good eye co-ordination; it is important to posses all the qualities outlined in the GMC guidelines about the duties of a doctor.

Pros: Extremely practical with hands-on approach; highly varied specialty; very rewarding (your efforts will be personally acknowledged by your satisfied patients); excellent opportunity to work in a multi-disciplinary team; challenging and expanding specialty; opportunity for research; has the potential for private practice for those interested.

Cons: Very competitive at entry level; busy on-call rota even as a consultant.

Sub-specialties: Trauma surgery; upper (further divided into shoulder, elbow, wrist and hand surgery) and lower (further divided into hip, knee, ankle and feet surgery) limb surgery, surgical procedures include joint replacement, arthroscopic surgery, ligament reconstruction and correction of congenital deformities; oncological surgery; spinal surgery (deals exclusively with traumatic, degenerative, neoplastic and congenital disorders of the spine).

Allied specialties: Plastic surgery; neurosurgery; accident & emergency; thoracic surgery; general surgery; intensive care; demonstrator of anatomy.

Royal College website address: England and Wales (www.rcseng.ac.uk); Edinburgh (www.rcsed.ac.uk); British Orthopaedic Society (www.boa.ac.uk); Welsh Orthopaedic Society (www.wos.ac).

Because of changes resulting from the *Modernising Medical Careers* (MMC) initiative (*see* Chapter 7), the time taken to become a consultant, and thus attain your ultimate career goal, is now relatively short. In addition, the MMC initiative has encouraged organisation of the career pathway of doctors. The improved career advice from sources such as this *Handbook*, specialised medical career advisers and medical career fairs (*see* Chapter 4), means there will be less confusion for potential and current doctors working in the NHS.

Lastly, revisit the usually stated reasons why it is good to work as a doctor in the NHS. You must have thought of some reasons why you wanted to become a doctor before you applied to medical school. Was it the job satisfaction, working with people who need your help, the status, the idea of making a difference to people's lives, the diversity and interests of various career pathways you can take, the achievements you gain along the way, the ability to work anywhere in the world, or just the big pay packet? From this, nowhere near exhaustive list, it is plain to see that there are plenty of reasons why it is desirable to be a doctor in the NHS. This perhaps explains why applications to medical school are always likely to remain high.

References

1   www.dh.gov.uk/PolicyAndGuidance/HumanResourcesAndTraining/ModernisingPay/
    JuniorDoctorContracts/JuniorDoctorContractsArticle/fs/en?CONTENT_ID=4053873&chk
    =77RU2U

2   Department of Health, National Assembly for Wales, NHS Confederation et al. *Guidance on
    Working Patterns for Junior Doctors*, 2002. (Available from www.dh.gov.uk/assetRoot/04/
    06/99/67/04069967.pdf)

3   Department of Health. *Improving Working Lives Standard*, 2000. (Available from
    www.dh.gov.uk/assetRoot/04/07/40/65/04074065.pdf)

4   www.rmbf.org

Further reading

Gray C. Life, your career and the pursuit of happiness. *BMJ Careers*. 1997: **315**: 2.

12

Postgraduate working conditions and pay

This chapter provides information about how your salary will be calculated, different ways you may work in the future, and advice on how to work shifts. It gives information about training schemes that help you to continue with your career under various circumstances. Finally, and, perhaps, most importantly, the chapter contains advice on how to maintain a good work–life balance.

Junior doctors' working conditions have been contentious for many years. Recently, there have been substantial changes to improve the working lives of junior doctors:

- in 2000 a new contract for junior doctors was drawn up
- in 2001 the maximum hours worked in a week for pre-registration house officers/ Foundation Year 1 doctors (PRHOs/F1s) was reduced to 56 hours
- by 2003 all junior doctors had a maximum limit of 56 working hours per week
- from August 2004 the European Working Time Directive (EWTD), an initiative designed to protect the health and safety of workers in the European Union, was applied to the medical profession[1]
- by 2009 all junior doctors will work a maximum of 48 hours, averaged over a reference period.[1]

The EWTD requires that trainee doctors have 11 hours' continuous rest in 24 hours; 24 hours' continuous rest in seven days (or 48 hours in 14 days); at least a 20-minute break every six hours; four weeks' annual leave and, for night workers, no more than eight hours' work in 24 hours, averaged over a reference period.[1]

The new contract did not leave junior doctors worse off but the EWTD has reduced their levels of pay and increased concerns about the amount of training junior doctors now receive. A positive effect of these reforms is that the working environment has been made less intense.

The salaries that junior doctors are paid relate to the hours worked and how antisocial the working hours are, as shown in Table 12.1. Based on these factors, levels of pay are organised into bands. A doctor will receive a basic salary plus a pay supplement (a percentage of the basic salary), based on the banding of that particular job.

Your post will be monitored every six months, and you will have to fill in diary cards, as a condition of your terms and conditions of service. If your post exceeds the hours or rest requirements then you may be put into Band 3; this means you will have a multiple of 100% of your basic salary. You should then work with your trust to ensure the rota becomes legal.

Table 12.1:   Description of pay banding and supplements for 2006

Antisocial	Explanation	Band 1: less than 48 hours/week[1]	Band 2: 48–56 hours/ week[1]	Band 3: more than 56 hours/ week[1]
Most	Resident on-call more than one in six Weekend more than one in three or more than one-third of hours worked outside 7 am to 7 pm Monday to Friday	50%	80%	Illegal
Moderate	Low intensity non-resident on-call More than one in eight weekends More often than one in four or more than one-third of hours worked outside 7 am to 7 pm Monday to Friday	40%	–	Illegal
Least	Low frequency non-resident on-call	20%	50%	Illegal

A rough guide to your future pay and the increments that co-exist with career progression will now be given. However, changes in working times may result in these being incorrect in the future.

The starting annual salary for Foundation 1 (F1) doctors in August 2005 was nearly £20,000.[2] This was the basic salary before including a banding supplement. A typical new doctor in a high-intensity post would therefore receive a minimum of £35,000 per annum.[2]

Foundation 2 (F2) doctors will earn the same as the first-year senior house officers (SHOs) who preceded them. That is, a basic annual salary of between £24,000 and £35,000, depending on how long they have been an SHO. An SHO in a typical high-intensity post can earn around £50,000 per annum after banding supplements have been added.[2]

Specialist registrars earn a basic salary of between £27,000 and £42,000, which increases to £60,007 per annum after supplements have been added for a typical high-intensity post.[2]

GP registrars receive the same basic salary as they earned in their last hospital training post. On top of this a 65% supplement is added.[2] Therefore a GP registrar who has previously been in hospital training posts for three years may earn around £46,000 per year.[2]

Consultants earn a basic salary between £67,000 and £91,000 per annum but may receive out-of-hours supplements and clinical excellence awards. Such awards may be worth an additional £69,000, for a Platinum award, but, realistically, only very few will achieve this.[2]

Most GPs are self-employed, though some are salaried. An average full-time, self-employed GP may earn at least £72,000 per annum[3] and often up to £120,000 per annum.

Pensions

All NHS contracted staff may enter the NHS pension scheme.[3] Within this scheme you make payments amounting to 6% of your salary, to which the NHS adds the equivalent of 14% of your salary.[3] In 2006, the entitlement is that your pension, when you retire, is 1/80th of your final salary for each full year you work in the NHS.[3] When you retire you may also receive a tax-free lump sum worth up to three times your annual pension, however, you should check this out when you start working as this may change.[3] Thus the NHS pension compares well to other non-health pension schemes.

Private practice

The NHS was founded in 1948 to provide healthcare, free at the point of use. Since the creation of the NHS, the private sector has become relatively small, with only 11% of the population having private healthcare insurance.[4]

For GPs there is no limit on receiving income through private practice and commercial contracts, provided NHS commitments are met.[4] However, if NHS premises are used, and more than 10% of the money earned by the practice is through non-NHS work, the primary care trust will proportionally reduce the reimbursements to the practice.[4]

Consultants have no restriction on their private earnings under the new consultant contract.[4] They must only demonstrate that they are fulfilling their NHS job plan, and there must be no conflict of interest between NHS work and private practice work.[4]

For junior doctors and staff-grade doctors there is also no limit on private practice provided that the private work is done outside contracted hours and does not interfere with their duties.[4]

Your trust, who is your main employer, is entitled to know of any work you carry out outside your normal contracted hours. It is entitled to prohibit you from other employment if it is felt that this interferes with the service you give to the trust.

Trusts are also entitled to know if you are doing extra locums; you may be prohibited from doing these if they interfere with your training, or trust service.

Private hospitals will not give admitting rights to anyone but those on the Specialist Register. Your NHS indemnity will not cover any other form of private activity so you will need to arrange additional, private indemnity insurance.

Junior doctors, including GP registrars, should seek the agreement of the relevant consultant or GP trainer, before doing any private practice.[4] Realistically, permission would rarely be granted as extra work is likely to impinge on doctors' capacity to learn and develop in their training posts.

A controversial issue with private practice is the perceived 'queue jumping' by private patients. The truth is that British patients may opt into or out of NHS-funded treatment at any stage.[4] However, patients who have had a private consultation initially, but then re-enter NHS-funded treatment, should be placed at the same position on the waiting list as if their original consultation had been within the NHS.[5] Although the General Medical Council (GMC) allows doctors to advertise their services publicly it is unethical to spend time discussing or promoting private practice during NHS consultations.[5]

Locum work

Locum doctors are 'stand-in' doctors, who cover the work of permanent doctors who are sick, on annual leave or away from work for any other reason. Locums can also be appointed to cover a position that has not yet been filled. You can only work as a locum if you are qualified to the degree that is required by the position you are 'stepping into'. You must also be covered by appropriate indemnity insurance.

If you have a full-time NHS post, your trust is entitled to know if you are doing extra locum sessions.

To work as a locum doctor in hospital or general practice, you may wish to register with a locum agency or you can be employed directly; remuneration from each source of work may be different, and you will have to investigate this to get the best deal. You can register with as many agencies as you wish and you have no commitments until you accept a locum position. The positive points about locum work are that you:

- know how much and how often you will receive your money once the work is arranged
- can work flexibly – not tied down to a contract
- can work in the location you desire
- can earn money whilst planning a career change, travel, etc.

The negative points about locum work include:

- an unpredictable income
- no paid study leave or annual leave
- no chance to familiarise yourself with a hospital
- it usually does not count towards training
- having to become familiar with the requirements of being self-employed (e.g. Income Tax, National Insurance, keeping accounts), if you are working in general practice (unless you are employed by an agency).

To work as a GP locum you need to be on an NHS trust performers' list.

Shift work

Working horrendous shifts was once seen as a rite of passage into the upper ranks of the medical profession. Doctors used to work a normal day and then remain on-call through the night or weekend.[6] This caused disruption to their circadian rhythms, resulting in daytime sleepiness and fatigue.

Rotational shifts are a good way of organising shift work. The best rotating shift is the fast-forward rotation.[6] An example of this shift pattern is to work two mornings then two afternoons and then two nights. The worst shift pattern is the opposite, the backward-rotating shift. This would involve, for example, a week of nights then a week of afternoons then a week of mornings.

Shift work, especially at night, has many negative effects on junior doctors, which include:[6]

- disruption of the normal circadian rhythm
- 'shift lag' – short-term sleepiness, insomnia, digestive problems and reduced mental agility
- significant effects on performance – studies of practical ability and efficiency show significant dips occur between 10 pm and 6 am, with a trough at 3 am[6]

- sleep disturbance
- loss of rapid eye movement during sleep.

The physical risks of shift work include:[6]

- peptic ulcer disease
- coronary heart disease
- miscarriage, low birth weight and pre-term birth
- injury – injury is more likely to occur during night shifts compared to day shifts.

The risks and effects of shift work illustrate the importance of learning how to protect your health while working shifts, especially night shifts. Here are a few tips to help you when you are working night shifts:[6]

- take short breaks every hour
- only drink coffee in the first half of the shift
- take a main meal break between midnight and 1 am – eat a protein-rich or health food
- take a smaller food break between 3 am and 4 am
- take naps to reduce sleepiness but be aware of sleep inertia: a period of reduced alertness 5–15 minutes after waking
- avoid driving to or from work
- eat healthily and stay fit
- avoid shift work if you are pregnant.

Specialty profile: Paediatrics

| 5 years | (M) | /+++\ |

Name: Dr Helen Goodyear
Position: Consultant Paediatrician
Hospital: Heart of England NHS Foundation Trust, Birmingham
Daily activities: There is not really a typical day. We do a week at a time as 'on-take consultant of the week' where all sessions are related to acute clinical care; this is enjoyable but exhausting, in particular in the winter season where over 40 admissions per day are common, including very sick children. The day begins with an hour's administration, signing reports and letters, dealing with general correspondence and e-mails. Clinic is at 9 am, which (it is hoped) is finished by 1 pm, including letters. We have regular lunchtime meetings. In the afternoon I see patients on the ward, referred for my special interest of paediatric dermatology. I also teach students, perform senior house officer assessments, attend various committees or planning groups, child strategy meetings or conferences and deal with the day's post and e-mails. I often need to phone parents; either to return their call, to give them results or arrange meetings with them for more complex cases.
Qualities required: Must like children and not just babies; be a team worker; have patience; have the ability to listen to both parents and children, and adapt what you are saying so that both can understand; flexibility of approach; good manual dexterity.
Pros: Most children come into hospital unwell but get better quickly and go home; friendly teamworking; great variety.

Cons: More paperwork and less clinical work the more senior that you get; on-call commitments are high even as a senior consultant; emotionally tough when a child dies.

Sub-specialties: There are some recognised sub-specialties but having a special interest is almost essential for most general paediatricians. However, there are a limited number of posts for tertiary specialists so many find employment as general paediatricians with a special interest.

Allied specialties: General practice; accident and emergency; critical care. Doing your elective abroad, in a developing country: seeing a different aspect of child health; undertaking a paediatric project. Voluntary work with children, there is a wide range possible here so that you are sure that you like being with children. Get a general paediatric student selected component just so that you know what it is like on a paediatric ward. They tend to be much noisier than adult wards. Join the acute admitting team for the week and you will get lots of exposure to children, which is different to when being taught.

Royal College website address: www.rcpch.ac.uk

Sleep disturbance is the most common effect of shift work. Tips to deal with this include:[6]

- ensure the room you sleep in is quiet and darkened
- avoid caffeine, smoking, alcohol and sleeping pills
- some people find taking melatonin before trying to sleep helps (consult appropriately trained health professionals before trying this).

The EWTD requires employers to assess the health of shift workers free of charge and at regular intervals. This is usually done using a questionnaire that is completed every three years for those under the age of 45 years and every two years for those over the age of 45 years.

Flexible working

Flexible training scheme

The flexible training scheme allows doctors to work 'less than full-time' in posts that are fully recognised for training and have the educational approval of the Postgraduate Medical Education and Training Board (PMETB) by recommendation of the postgraduate deaneries and royal colleges.[7] Flexible training posts are available for doctors who are unable to train full-time for good reasons.

There are four types of flexible training placements:[7]

- Flexible/supernumerary posts – additional to the normal complement of trainees in a particular specialty.
- Part-time working reduced hours in a full-time slot (applies mainly to specialist registrars) – a trainee reduces the hours they work, for example having a full weekday off, working half days or having flexible start and finish times.
- Slot share – two flexible trainees cover the duties of a full-time post. Each post should include between 50% and 70% of full-time hours and last for 6 or 12 months. Slot share partners may change depending on individual training needs.

- Job-share – a training placement is divided between two trainees. The two trainees cover all the original duties of a full-time post. No eligibility criteria is required if the employer is satisfied that the jobsharers are the best candidates at appointment. The two candidates must send in a joint application, plan how to work together to obey their contractual obligations and decide how they will divide annual/study leave and pay.

The associate dean for flexible training decides at a confidential meeting whether or not a candidate's reasons are well founded and thus whether or not they receive the flexible training post.[7] Candidates who apply for a flexible training post can be divided into two categories, based on the reasons they give for applying.[7]

Category 1

Candidates who have been professionally disadvantaged by their circumstances and are less able to fulfil their potential when working full-time, for reasons such as:

- disability or ill-health
- responsibility for children (doctor of either gender)
- caring for an ill or disabled partner, relative or other dependant.

Category 2

- unique opportunities for personal/professional development
- service to the wider NHS
- other reasons.

Only in exceptional circumstances would undertaking research be considered a reason for flexible training, as it should be accommodated within the ordinary training programme.

Category 1 applicants are usually funded and chosen for flexible training posts in preference to Category 2 applicants.[7] However, when funds are limited all the applicants will be placed in order of priority for funding and occasionally a Category 2 applicant may be chosen in preference to a Category 1 applicant.[7] Factors that may influence the candidate's priority for funding include:[7]

- their specialty
- duration of funding; for example, trainees near the end of their training may require a shorter duration of funding than other trainees
- the candidate being able to display commitment or progress
- available funding.

If a trainee moves to another deanery a flexible post will not be funded automatically.[7]

The appointment process differs among different grades of trainees. F1 doctors apply via the multi-deanery appointment process for a Foundation Programme in exactly the same way as a full-timer. A flexible post may then be arranged following successful application.[7]

Foundation Year 2 doctors either apply for flexible posts in the deanery or arrange for flexible training after getting a F2 post.[7]

For SHO and specialist registrars who want flexible training, the process of applying for a training post is exactly the same as for those who want to train full-time.[7] The best candidate is offered the job but for the flexible trainee, funding, educational approval, work hours and the agreement of the trust and deanery to accept a flexible trainee must be organised before they start their job.[7]

All flexible trainees must work a minimum of 50% of a full-time post at their trust.[7] GP vocational training scheme (VTS) trainees must complete one week of full-time training during hospital placements and in the GP registrar year.[7] Trainees must not work more than 40 hours per week unless they are working reduced hours in a full-time slot.[7] Like full-time training posts there are payment bands for flexible trainees:[7]

- Band FA: 50% supplement – high intensity and most antisocial hours.
- Band FB: 40% supplement – moderate intensity and fewer antisocial hours.
- Band FC: 20% supplement – trainees with duties outside the period 7 am to 7 pm Monday to Friday.

No supplement is paid if all the hours are between 7 am and 7 pm Monday to Friday and are less than 40 hours per week.

Specialty profile: Pathology

| 4–5 years | L | + |

Name: Dr Paul Matthews
Position: Consultant Histopathologist, Honorary Senior Lecturer
Hospital: University Hospitals Coventry and Warwickshire, Walsgrave Hospital, Coventry
Daily activities: Working a rota system with eight other histopathologists, I am responsible for the preparation of complex surgical resection specimens, reporting on histological specimens large and small, reporting on cytological specimens, carrying out autopsies and contributing to multi-disciplinary meetings. I also run modules in Phase 1 and 2 of the Warwick University Medical School graduate entry course. Any one day may involve several or all of these duties, not forgetting some audit and research. Other days might include interviewing prospective medical students or giving evidence at Coroner's Court. I work as part of a team within the department of pathology (e.g. technicians, laboratory staff, secretaries) and as part of clinical teams managing patient care.
Qualities required: A degree of obsessional behaviour; ability to communicate well both verbally and in written form; ability to know your skills and limitations (I often ask a colleague for an opinion); ability to assimilate information from many sources; ability to do three jobs at once (on a quiet day).
Pros: Time to think (unless it's during a frozen section); flexibility to do routine work around other commitments (like answering this questionnaire!); getting close to the elusive, absolute right answer to the question 'What is going wrong with this patient?' (sometimes not possible); working closely with clinicians who listen very closely to what you have to say; a pathologist's opinion may decide whether someone has a radical procedure or toxic chemotherapy; ability to combine routine work with medical school commitments; rarely called in at night.
Cons: Loss of direct patient contact; public perceptions that you only do autopsy work; hardly a glamour specialty; getting very much busier.

Sub-specialties: Almost all pathologists specialise now and have responsibility for one or more sub-specialties. For example, I have an interest in lymphomas and head and neck pathology. Forensics appeals to some while others forsake autopsy work altogether. Some generalisation still happens though. For example, today I have made diagnoses on biopsies from lymph node, tongue, pleura, colon and salivary gland. Variety remains the spice of life.

Allied specialty: Job-wise nothing is a substitute for an F2 post in histopathology. Any clinical experience is a bonus for pathology and any clinical job would benefit from a time in pathology. Go to the mortuary for teaching on clinical aspects of pathology. Follow your patient's biopsy. Seek an elective in pathology, not necessarily in the UK. Turn up for multi-disciplinary meetings and see how pathologists contribute to patient management. Badger a pathologist to run a Special Study Module!

Royal College website address: www.rcpath.org

Flexible Careers Scheme

The Flexible Careers Scheme[8] allows consultants, GPs and hospital doctors of all grades to work up to 50% of full-time.[8] The scheme was developed to provide doctors with an opportunity to work flexibly whilst being supported in maintaining their career.[8] The range of doctors who use this scheme include those who want to work less than 50% of full-time, those who are, or will soon be, retired and those who want to return to work in medicine but need a period of supervised work.[8]

Until 2005, NHS Professionals were responsible for the Flexible Careers Scheme, working in partnership with local postgraduate deaneries in England.[8] The scheme could be adapted to suit individual needs and provided enough clinical practice for revalidation purposes.[8] There was a limit to how long a person could stay on the Flexible Careers Scheme but extensions were possible.[8] At the end of 2005, the funding for the scheme was devolved by the Department of Health to local NHS organisations. The available funding proved inadequate to support the numbers of doctors wishing to access the scheme. At the time of writing, it remains unclear as to how the scheme will be managed and resourced in the future. This is a great shame, considering how successful it has been in the past.

Work–life balance

Research has shown that there are three types of hospital consultant in terms of work–life balance. These types are described based on the relation between their career and their personal or family lives.[9]

- Career-dominant:
  - characteristics: single, divorced, childless
  - career course: full-time, continuous
  - reflections: female – some made a conscious decision not to have a family; both males and females – some expressed strong regrets about neglecting their lives outside medicine.

- Segregated:
  - characteristics: married/divorced, with/without children, family responsibilities organised to enable more time to be involved in their career
  - career course: full-time, continuous
  - reflections: male – many dissatisfied with their work–life balance and blame pressure to conform to intensive work practices; female – many believed this approach was the only way to achieve consultant grades and have a family.
- Accommodating:
  - characteristics: married/cohabiting, children
  - career course: males – full-time, continuous; females – career break and/or periods of part-time training/work
  - reflections: both males and females expressed satisfaction with their work–life balance.[9]

In order for you to achieve your perfect balance of working towards and within a career in medicine, and living a life outside medicine, you must think about:[10]

- your own definition of happiness
- your perfect day in the future
- how you will get to your perfect life.

You must also think about how you will cope with the risks to your standard of living that come with a career in medicine, for example:[11]

- high prevalence of stress
- discordance between public image and realities of your job
- low morale
- high divorce rate
- high risk of substance and alcohol abuse.

A tip to assist you with contemplating your ideal work–life balance is to devise a life strategy with goals. You should think about the path to reach your goals as well as any obstacles you may face both in your work and personal lives.[11]

When you are working as a doctor, managing your work–life balance will initially involve thinking about the purpose of your life and its importance to others. You should reflect on your current work–life balance and what areas of your life you may be neglecting.[12] A good way of doing this is to list eight roles that you occupy (including your role as your own body's carer), and then rate how well you fulfil those roles on a scale of one to ten.[12] Not only will this provide you with an overview of your life you will easily see if you are neglecting any role.[12] You can then direct your energy towards the roles that require increased attention and improved performance.

In order to be happy whilst working in medicine it is important to remain fit and spend enough time concentrating on non-medical things. You should deal promptly with any problems as they arise. Problems can occur in many areas of your non-medical life, and you should monitor your health, finances, relationships and social life, in order to pick up difficulties early on.[11]

Help with managing your work–life balance is available from the Royal Medical Benevolent Fund (RMBF). The RMBF website (www.support4doctors.org) is an independent and non-judgemental source of support that includes:[11]

- information on how to find different sources of support, for example information on careers, finance, health and family life
- contact details for peer support telephone helplines
- information on achieving a good work–life balance.

References

1   Department of Health. *Guidance on Working Patterns for Junior Doctors*, 2002. (Available from www.dh.gov.uk/assetRoot/04/06/99/67/04069967.pdf)

2   British Medical Association. *Doctor's and Dentist's Review Body Report*, 2005. (Available from www.bma.org.uk/ap.nsf/content/DDRB2005summary)

3   National Health Service. *Pay and Benefits*, 2005. (Available from www.nhscareers.nhs.uk/nhs-knowledge_base/data/5340.html)

4   British Medical Association. *Fees for Part-time Medical Service*, 2004. (Available from www.bma.org.uk/ap.nsf/Content/feesparttimemed_privatepractice?OpenDocument Highlight+2,private,practice)

5   British Medical Association. *Interface Between NHS and Private Treatment*, 2004. (Available from www.bma.org.uk/ap.nsf/Content/NHSprivate)

6   Hobson J. Shift work and doctors' health. *BMJ Career Focus*. 2004; **329**: 149–50.

7   West Midlands Deanery. *Flexible Careers and Training*. (Available from www.wmdeanery.org/careerguide/flextraining.asp)

8   Department of Health. *Flexible Working for Doctors Highlighted*, 2003. (Available from www.dh.gov.uk/PublicationsAndStatistics/PressReleases/PressReleasesNotices/fs/en?CONTENT_ID=4047391&chk=cf9LHu)

9   Dumelow C, Littlejohns P and Griffiths S. Relation between a career and family for English hospital consultants: qualitative semi-structured interview study. *BMJ*. 2000; **320**: 1437–40.

10 Steel N. Planning your life and career. *BMJ Career Focus*. 1999; **319**: 2.

11 Gray C. Life, your career and the pursuit of happiness. *BMJ Careers*. 1997; **315**: 2.

12 Houghton A. Personal support 3: how to help someone achieve balance in their working and personal lives. *BMJ Career Focus*. 2005; **331**: 7–8.

Further reading

BMA website (www.bma.org.uk).

13

Preparation for future jobs

> This chapter provides general advice for you to use when you are preparing to apply for jobs at any stage of your career. Consider the advice given here in conjunction with Chapter 9.

Record of professional development

It is never too early to start preparing for future jobs. The earlier you start the better. One way of preparing for job applications is by using a record of professional development (ROPD). Official ROPD folders are handed out in some medical schools to students in their pre-clinical years. If this does not happen at your medical school, you can easily create your own by buying a large ring binder or box file and some dividers.

The purpose of a ROPD is to collate information about your skills, achievements and interests. It is a record of proof to support what you have been doing throughout your training and career to date. You can then either take the whole thing to future interviews or use it to create a personal summary.

Information contained within your ROPD should include:

- a regularly updated CV (*see below*)
- summary of exam, project and assessment results
- copies of written projects, reports and published papers
- regularly updated career aspirations, strengths and weaknesses, and current views on your professional development; you could use the forms in appendices 2 and 3, designed for this purpose
- details of skills you have which are relevant to professional development.

Set aside some time on a regular basis – maybe each time you get exam results – to go through your ROPD and update each section. It is easy to forget about relevant information if you do not complete this until the end of your medical training. It does not take long to keep your ROPD up to date and it will be incredibly useful to you. Carry on the collation of this information in your postgraduate career. The key to a successful ROPD is that it is contemporary and accurate.

Specialist and general practice training programmes

The specialist and general practice training programme[1] application process is competitive, just like that for Foundation posts. The selection process utilises information and evidence gathered during your Foundation Programme.

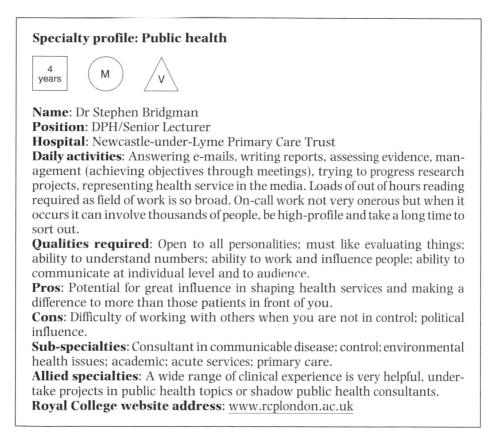

Specialty profile: Public health

Name: Dr Stephen Bridgman
Position: DPH/Senior Lecturer
Hospital: Newcastle-under-Lyme Primary Care Trust
Daily activities: Answering e-mails, writing reports, assessing evidence, management (achieving objectives through meetings), trying to progress research projects, representing health service in the media. Loads of out of hours reading required as field of work is so broad. On-call work not very onerous but when it occurs it can involve thousands of people, be high-profile and take a long time to sort out.
Qualities required: Open to all personalities; must like evaluating things; ability to understand numbers; ability to work and influence people; ability to communicate at individual level and to audience.
Pros: Potential for great influence in shaping health services and making a difference to more than those patients in front of you.
Cons: Difficulty of working with others when you are not in control; political influence.
Sub-specialties: Consultant in communicable disease; control; environmental health issues; academic; acute services; primary care.
Allied specialties: A wide range of clinical experience is very helpful, undertake projects in public health topics or shadow public health consultants.
Royal College website address: www.rcplondon.ac.uk

Application and selection onto these further training programmes occurs prior to the end of your Foundation years. Contrary to some beliefs, you do not have to have done a Foundation post in the exact field in which you want to specialise. It is expected that you have gained some experience in related or relevant areas. The various specialty profiles throughout this book should assist you with finding allied areas to gain experience. The *Modernising Medical Careers* (MMC) initiative supports the development of career counselling throughout medical school and your Foundation years. This should help you decide which specialist programme suits you best. Look at the relevant Royal College websites to gain more information on the training programmes of individual specialties (*see* Appendix 4).

Recent changes to the application process to GP training schemes have resulted in a standardised and consistent online electronic system. Much like the online application process for many Foundation Programme applications, the GP training application consists of online registration and application forms. Applicants are able to indicate their deanery of preference and track the progress of their application.

Curriculum vitae

Your curriculum vitae[2-6] (CV) is incredibly important. Despite the current trend of scoring systems and structured application forms for postgraduate job applications, CVs are often a major part of the contact you make when applying for jobs. In addition, the number of applicants to postgraduate posts is increasing.[7] It is crucial that your CV is accurate, current and gives a fantastic first impression.

Although there is not a standard format, presentation or type of CV that will impress everyone,[7] the presentation and content can influence the chances of a successful application.

The first tip is *do not lie*. You must be ready to be asked about every single thing you write in your CV. If you are audited and found to be lying you may risk your registration with the General Medical Council (GMC).

When writing your CV, an important and useful starting point is to follow any instructions present in the job advertisement. Although obvious, this is not always done and can be a way for recruiters to weed out the first set of CVs for rejection.[7]

Nowadays it is expected that your CV is wordprocessed and printed on good quality paper. The use of a laser printer to print your CV is recommended; however, if you do not have one of these it is not necessary to use a professional company to produce your CV. Just ensure, before you send it off, that there are no smudges. Tabulation, especially of qualifications and personal details, allows quick and easy reference. CVs that lack clarity, have an unstructured layout and are not easy to read do not impress the recruitment team; factors such as these may result in an immediate rejection of your application regardless of the content.[7]

You must include information such as training and experience in specific and/or relevant areas to the job you are applying for. Often experience gained within posts is assumed; highlight anything particularly special or outstanding about any aspect of your particular job.[7] For example, if you have worked in the country's leading liver unit with a highly renowned hepatologist, point this out, otherwise someone may assume you worked in the gastroenterology department in a small district general hospital.

In apparent contrast to the above, it is important that you do not just include information narrowly involved with the specialty to which you are applying. Try and think a bit more laterally and include details of your experience and skills in allied specialties. You may wish to include work within varying populations, highlighting your broad clinical experience. Conversely, if your previous experience has not been directly related to the job you should clearly justify how it is relevant to the post you are applying for. Your application will not be dismissed if you can prove that previous unrelated positions are not due to a failure in your career progression or indecisiveness (*see* Box 13.1).

Box 13.1: Suggested information for inclusion in your CV

Curriculum vitae

Personal details:

- Names (first name(s), surname)
- Your main or most recent qualification
- GMC registration number, valid training permit, experience in the UK
- Postal address
- Telephone (landline and/or mobile), e-mail and fax (where applicable)
- Date of birth, age

Career details:

- Education:
  - qualifications, prizes, relevant non-academic achievements – GCSE/A-levels (or equivalent) become irrelevant, university degrees and grades are essential; BMedSci is less relevant if obtained through an integrated medical degree unless it resulted in first-class honours or a publication
  - courses
  - dates
  - institution and location
- Work history – in reverse chronological order – and can include elective, research and relevant part-time jobs (e.g. healthcare assistant, GP note summariser):
  - date
  - position
  - current employer's name and location
  - duties, achievements and experience – think about the following areas: leadership; self-motivation and initiative; time management; teamwork; teaching; communicating with patients and professional colleagues; other than in surgery or anaesthetics, listing specific procedures you have performed is unnecessary, if applying for surgery or anaesthetics you should ensure you have an up-to-date log book to refer to
- Published work – holds more weight if published in reputable journal, quality>quantity
- Clinical audit and research – valued equally, often only count if resulting in publication
- Courses and conferences you have attended:
  - dates
  - location
  - name
- Presentations you have given
- Career aspirations:
  - brief statement – it may not be definitive in junior doctor years
  - include how you think the job will help you to achieve these aspirations

Additional information and useful skills:

- Clinical
- Computer
- Languages
- Management – this is not necessary as a junior doctor; however, it is a bonus
- Administration

Personal specification:

- Interests
- Desirable criteria – aspects of professional or personal life you are proud of
- Leisure activities

Referees – usually you require two, it is polite to ask permission first:

- Names – one should be your current boss; well-known or distinguished names can be good if possible
- Postal address
- Telephone, e-mail and fax (where applicable)

As a medical student looking ahead at this chapter you are in an advantageous position because you have the time to plan and adhere to the advice being given. You can also ensure you work hard at preventing gaps appearing in your career pathway. However, gaps may be unavoidable, and for the junior doctors reading this, they may have already occurred. To prevent these gaps holding you back you must be able to justify them appropriately when applying for future jobs. Depending on the reason for the gaps, you may be able to relate the experiences you gained during that time, or the problems you were having, to you being a better applicant now.

Any work in progress may be included on your CV, but exercise caution: work in progress may be interpreted as your inability to finish anything, or something that will interfere with the performance of your next post. Present your work in progress to demonstrate that you are a hive of activity and have constantly got something on the go. If you can show that there is an exciting piece of work that has not reached its conclusion at the time of the CV application, you may be asked about it at interview.

Try hard to think of appropriate and useful qualities and experience you have, which other applicants may not have. These may include projects, part-time jobs or voluntary work. You should aim to demonstrate an appropriate level of knowledge and experience. However, it is important that you can prove you are a well-rounded and a potentially invaluable member of the team.

Box 13.1 illustrates the type of information recommended for inclusion in your CV. This is a full illustration, demonstrating many aspects you may like to include but very few people, especially early on in their career, will be able to write something under every heading. If all headings can be filled, your CV will probably be too long. Pick out the most important and relevant points to match the job specifications. Number the pages for ease of reference at an interview. Bear in mind, this is a highly personal document, so add in anything else you think is relevant and feel free to personalise the design of your CV. If you are unsure about the inclusion of certain personal information, ask senior colleagues for advice. You may also require advice from a medico-legal company depending on what your query is.

A word of warning: do not let your artistic temperament take over so much that your CV loses its professionalism. Consultants and others involved in recruiting you may not see your new-found favourite font in bright pink as 'cool' or 'funky' but more as 'strange', 'juvenile' or 'pathetic'. However, some people may use colour or include a photo in order to make their CV stand out. You will have to consider the use of such things critically in each case.

Finally, before you send off your CV, check it for errors in spelling, grammar and formatting. Although useful, computer spelling and grammar-checking functions are not foolproof; for example, they do not pick up errors in spellings that have resulted in a wrong but recognised word. Use an A4 envelope to prevent excessive creases in the document. Your CV will be more striking if it is a crisp, crease-free sheet.

Interview skills[8–11]

Interviews provoke a reaction that is closely related to fear and terror in most people. Therefore, let us start on a positive note: if your application has reached the stage that you have been called for interview you have already impressed your potential employers. You can be safe in the knowledge that the information they have received from you so far has satisfied the basic requirements for the job.

So why do they need to see you? The two main aims of the interview process are:

- to confirm whether you have the required professional competencies
- to find out whether they think you would be a good colleague; that is, they want to explore your personality and attitudes.

The most important things you can think about before an interview are preparation and personal presentation.

Preparation

Preparation is key. Ever heard the old adage 'Fail to prepare, prepare to fail'? Nowhere is this more relevant. Do not attempt to go to an interview without prior preparation. Preparation for your interview requires just as much attention as the earlier stages of your application. Preparation and accumulation of relevant knowledge enables you to feel and appear more confident.

You have probably already submitted a fair amount of information either via an application form or your CV, or both. You should be able to explain, in detail, everything you have included in these documents. Take a copy so that you can refer the interviewers to the relevant sections in answer to questions – they may not have had time to read them in detail.

Areas in which it is a good idea to do prior research include the following.

- The actual job and your potential role in that job. You could:
    - contact people in the department
    - contact the person currently in the job you are applying for
    - find out about the bulk of the work in terms of conditions encountered and procedures performed
    - determine which proficiencies and skills are required for the job and, if you do not possess them, whether training for these occurs in the post
    - recent, relevant journals
    - 'hot topics' in the news, relevant to the job or specialty you are applying for
    - influential past and present research in the relevant specialty

- broad knowledge of the health service, including current debates and forth-coming developments.
- Questions, especially obvious ones, are a common area in which lack of preparation presents a major stumbling block in an interview. Although you do not want to rehearse the answers word-for-word, prepare rough answers for the most predictable questions. Some of these, and some advice regarding the answers, may include:
    - 'Why do you want the job?' – do not just mention pay, no overtime, good-looking nurses, etc.
    - 'Why do you want to work in this hospital or practice?' – think about the experiences provided by the service that interest you
    - 'What qualities do you have which you could bring to the job?' – 'Someone to have a good night out with,' will not impress the interview panel, no matter how young they are
    - 'Where do you see yourself, career-wise, in the future/in 5 years/in 10 years?'
    - 'What are your biggest achievements?' – these can be career- or non-career-related
    - 'How do you manage stress?' – the better applicants will not mention alcohol
    - 'What are research and audit? What are the differences between the two?'
    - 'What is clinical governance?' – this is a 'hot topic' and it is important you understand at least the basics of it
    - 'How would you describe your personality?' – highlight traits useful to the job
    - 'What are your strengths?' – use the forms in appendices 2 and 3 to assist in your answers to this question and the next one
    - 'What are your weaknesses?' – try not to use 'being a perfectionist', it is a common, boring and predictable answer to which an interviewer's equally boring and predictably response will be 'What is your second weakness?'
    - 'Do you have any questions?' – do not ask too many, but areas you may consider are: the particular clinical or research interests of the consultant or department; opportunities to gain experience in areas of particular interest to you; nature of senior on-call support; educational, study and training sessions provided.

Personal presentation

Advice on personal presentation for an interview encompasses behavioural and aesthetic aspects.

First impressions really do count. You do not want to be late, so leave plenty of time for your journey, getting lost and finding somewhere to park. Ensure that your mobile phone is switched off. When you enter the room, despite how you may be feeling, try to appear confident, with a warm smile. Offer a handshake when being introduced to each interviewer.

Be polite at all times. This includes not making any jokes which have the potential to offend anyone, even slightly. Ensure that you sit upright and that your posture (and answers) portrays openness and honesty. This may include not crossing your legs. Try not to fiddle with anything and keep your hand gestures contained and to a minimum. When answering questions ensure that you look around at the whole panel and try to gain good eye contact if your interviewers will engage in this.

Consider your choice of outfit. Men should always wear a suit or smart jacket and trousers. A tie is essential and comic ties have no place. Women should wear suits or at least a smart, matching jacket, but do not have to wear skirts. Smart trousers or dresses are acceptable. Neither gender should be wearing clothes with logos or slogans. Be comfortable with what you are wearing so you are not tempted to adjust items of clothing during the interview.

Your overall look should be clean, tidy and well groomed. Avoid bright colours in your hair, polish your shoes and do a final check for hanging threads, laddered tights or labels hanging out the back of the garments you are wearing.

How to deal with rejection[12]

Unfortunately rejection is common during a career in medicine. It can occur in response to attempts at publication, ideas for development as well as after job applications. This situation is not set to change in the near future, as more applicants are being rejected due to increasing numbers of applications for posts in the UK.

Everybody deals with rejection differently. Common feelings following rejection include negative emotions, such as sadness, anger and frustration, reduced motivation and doubts about self and career, perhaps leading to affected performance in your current job. None of these responses are problematic unless you experience them for a prolonged period of time. However, if negativity persists it may lead to depression, financial problems and further career problems. Haq and Agell[12] suggest the following practical steps to assist you with dealing with rejection.

- Share your feelings – a problem shared is not always a problem halved; however, sharing your feelings with other people opens up the opportunity for them to give advice. They may have been in a similar situation or be able to provide you with a different perspective, which may help you view your situation more positively.
- Seek advice from your mentor (*see* Chapter 5) or senior colleagues.
- Remind yourself of your strengths; the 'Current career interests' form in Appendix 2 will help you. You may have been rejected on only minor points. As you are good at many things, you should concentrate on these skills and abilities at times when you are feeling low in self-esteem.
- Assess whether or not your negative emotions are leading to depression. Seek help if you, or your friends or colleagues, are concerned.
- Prepare for financial problems in advance, decide upon a strategy in case of rejection before the application process begins.

Lastly, there are various support groups open to you. You may find a source of support internally through the trust you belong to or through external support groups, like the Doctors' Support Network. This provides an independent, friendly and supportive service run by volunteer doctors. (*See* Appendix 1 for contact details.)

International graduates and the 'PLAB test'

The Professional and Linguistic Assessments Board (PLAB) test is a two-part examination, set for non-European Economic Area (non-EEA) international graduates, in order to register with the GMC and compete for jobs in the UK.[13,14] The PLAB is designed to assess whether non-EEA international graduates have reached the minimum standard required in order to practise medicine safely in the UK.[13] Not all international graduates are required to take the PLAB, for example EEA graduates do not. It is up to each individual doctor to check with the GMC whether exemptions apply to them.[14]

You need more than successful PLAB results, if applicable, to register with the GMC. First, you must have an 'acceptable primary medical qualification'. Non-EEA international graduates must also demonstrate good English language skills (satisfactory scores on in the International English Language Testing System (IELTS)). Finally, graduates should have 12 months' postgraduate experience as a pre-registration house officer/Foundation Year 1 (PRHO/F1). Those without PRHO/F1 experience can still take the PLAB but would need to apply for an F1 job, for which the competition is exceedingly high.[13]

The PLAB test itself is divided into two parts. The first is a written paper containing 200 questions of two styles: extended matching questions (EMQs) and single best-answer questions (SBAs). SBA questions usually comprise no more than 30% of the paper. Part 2 is an objective structured clinical examination (OSCE) consisting of 14 five-minute stations. Although you may attempt Part 1 as many times as you wish, you must pass it within two years of passing your IELTS, when applicable. You may only take Part 2 four times and must pass this within three years of passing Part 1. If you fail four times you will be required to retake IELTS, if previously applicable, and Part 1 and Part 2 of the PLAB. Limited registration, from the GMC, must be granted within three years of successful completion of Part 2.

Passing the PLAB test does not automatically result in a job. In fact, because competition for jobs in the UK is so high, statistics show it takes at least six months to secure a job after passing the PLAB and many doctors do not have a job one year after. When accounting for the fees (over £500 for both PLAB tests plus the language exam), travel, visas and living costs, taking the PLAB test becomes very expensive.[13] The pass mark is set so that only a certain proportion of candidates pass at any one sitting. However, because the places are not rationed, many more people may take the PLAB test than there are medical posts.[13]

Useful experience can be gained by doctors in the UK by working on a clinical attachment. This is an unpaid post in which you can shadow a doctor. You can use this time to experience a specialty you have previously had an interest in to clarify whether or not it is for you, or you can use the time to familiarise yourself with NHS and hospital procedures (clinical and administrative).[13]

Delays in taking up a given post may occur even when international doctors have passed the PLAB test and been appointed. Hospital trusts may have to undertake checks with the criminal records bureau, and various health checks, before allowing overseas-graduate doctors access to their patients. They may also require additional insurance cover before a clinical attachment can be started, but this is up to individual hospitals to decide.

For more information on the PLAB test and the information provided here, please refer to www.gmc-uk.org. Here you will find further, up-to-date, information on what is involved, procedures and sample questions and scenarios to help you prepare for both parts of the examination.

Specialty profile: Radiology

| 5 years | H | ⚠ + |

Name: Dr Katharine Foster
Position: Paediatric Radiologist
Hospital: Birmingham Children's Hospital
Daily activities: I typically work from 9 am till 5 pm, but sometimes I have to arrive earlier for meetings and leave a bit later on other days. We have lists booked each day, so to some extent I know what my day is going to involve, but there are always inpatients and emergencies to be squeezed in. I do CT and plain films on Monday morning, fluoroscopy on Tuesday afternoon, CT and plain films on Wednesday morning, ultrasound Thursday morning and MRI all day Friday. The remaining time is spent at clinical meetings, teaching and catching up with reporting, and talking to other doctors in the hospital about scans and patients.
Qualities required: Fairly meticulous, organised but flexible, able to communicate with colleagues, families and children, a good memory helps, academic in that we spend quite a lot of time looking unusual conditions up in books.
Pros: I see lots of interesting patients but never have to tell them or their family bad news.
Cons: The radiology department is in many ways the centre of the hospital; people come down to see you all day to ask you about scans and patients.
Sub-specialties: Paediatric radiology is quite a specialised field already and at BCH we stay very general within that field, as everything needs to be covered on call. Some people have special interests, for example in musculoskeletal radiology. At Great Ormond Street there are more consultants, and hence more specialisation.
Allied specialty: Paediatrics!
Royal College website address: www.rcr.ac.uk

References

1 Department of Health. *Modernising Medical Careers: the next steps*, 2004. (Available from www.dh.gov.uk/assetRoot/04/07/95/32/04079532.pdf)

2 Houghton A. Getting that job: deciding to apply. *StudentBMJ*. 2003; **11**: 376.

3 McErin S. Writing a winning CV. *BMJ Career Focus*. 2004; **328**: 225.

4 Medical Forum. *CV Headings to Consider*. Available from www.medicalforum.com/cv-headings.htm)

5 Turya E. Growing your CV. *BMJ Career Focus*. 2004; **328**: 226.

6 Craft N. Making the shortlist. *BMJ Careers*. 1996; **313**: 2.

7 Ariyasena H, Tewari N and Livesley PJ. The search for the perfect curriculum vitae. *BMJ Career Focus*. 2005; **331**: 167–9.

8 Houghton A. Getting that job: preparing for interview. *StudentBMJ*. 2003; **11**: 414–15.

9   Sudlow M. How to be interviewed. *BMJ Careers.* 1996; **313**: 2.

10   Jewkes F. The advice zone. *BMJ Career Focus.* 2005; **331**: 64.

11   Thompson MJ and Heneghan C. Asking questions at the end of an interview for a clinical job. *BMJ Career Focus.* 2005; **331**: 67.

12   Haq SF and Agell I. Dealing with rejection. *BMJ Career Focus.* 2005; **331**: 75.

13   General Medical Council *Guidance for PLAB Test Candidates*, updated July 2005. (Available from www.gmc-uk.org/doctors/plab/Guidance_for_PLAB_test_candidates.pdf)

14   McGinn K and Haivas I. PLAB: key to the kingdom. *StudentBMJ.* 2005; **13**: 468–71.

Further reading

Agha R. *Making Sense of Your Medical Career: your strategic guide to success.* London: Hodder Arnold; 2005. (Appendix 2 of this book details some questions often asked at interview.)

British Medical Association. Overseas doctors: sink or swim. *BMJ Career Focus.* 2004. (Available from www.bmjcareers.com)

Burnett S. Dressing the part. *BMJ Career Focus.* 2005; **331**: 67.

Houghton A. Getting that job: the final offensive. *StudentBMJ.* 2003; **11**: 458.

Irish B. General practice: the bigger picture. *BMJ Career Focus.* 2005; **331**: 74. (Information for those considering a career in general practice.)

Poole A. What not to do at an interview. *BMJ Career Focus.* 2005; **331**: 65–6.

A survey of PLAB pass doctors may be found at www.gmc-uk.org

14

Research, academia and medical education in your career

Research, academia and medical education are crucial for the training of doctors and medical students as well as the progression of medicine as a whole. This chapter shows you how you can incorporate these three components into your career.

Research in your career

Research is performed in order to improve medical practice. You can take part in research at any point in your career. Examples of research opportunities include intercalated degrees, Foundation Year 2 (F2) academic jobs and case studies. Research is an important part of any modern health system that values evidence-based medicine.[1]

There are several good reasons for you to do research, including:[1]

- to improve your understanding of research techniques that will better enable you to critically interpret and understand published work
- to start a career-long involvement in research, either as a leader or as a member of a team
- as part of your training, for example to become an academic consultant.

If you are involved in research to complement what you foresee as a purely clinically role, it is sensible to focus on the specialty in which you wish to work.[1] If you intend to have a more academic career then the quality of the research is more important than the topic.[1]

Published research will enhance your CV, and thus your future job applications. After five years of working as a doctor, you may register with a university and submit a number of original pieces of work, for example a thesis and/or published papers, to be awarded a MD (doctor of medicine degree) or a PhD. Simply performing research does not automatically mean it will be published.[2] To increase the chances of getting your work published it should address a subject of interest to the editors (and readers) of the journals you decide to send it to and it must be of good quality.[2] Good research takes time, so you will require good time-management skills.[2]

The department in which you complete your research usually funds your studies. The department, in turn, receives financial support from research funding bodies or industry.[1] You can obtain funding from personal research training fellowships.[1]

These are more desirable and are awarded in open competition after peer review of a grant application that may be offered by the Medical Research Council (MRC), research charities or industry.[1]

Academic medicine in your career

To be a medical academic you must have an ongoing commitment to produce high quality research; not just a desire to increase the number of publications under your belt in order to improve your chances of being appointed as a consultant or an academic GP.[1] The *Modernising Medical Careers* (MMC) initiative is aiming to improve the training to become a medical academic.[2] There is no specific route into academic medicine.[1] It is a broad area of medicine in which most practitioners also work as clinicians or medical educators. Traditionally, doctors wishing to become academics usually have to train for longer than their non-academic colleagues.[3] As a result of the new F2 posts, and dedicated higher specialist training in academic medicine, the time spent as a junior medical academic should now be shorter.

The report, *Medically and Dentally Qualified Academic Staff: Recommendations for Training the Researchers and Educators of the Future,*[4] highlights previous barriers to pursuing an academic career in medicine and identifies ways to enter academia using 'an integrated clinical academic career pathway'. Specific recommendations, for medical students through to consultants, have been made to overcome the previous problems with a career in academic medicine. As the recommendations and new training pathways are implemented there will be increased support for anybody wanting to enter academic medicine during any stage in their career.

Medical education in your career

As with other academic medicine, there is no specific career route into medical education. To assist your career path in becoming a medical educator you can undertake various courses to improve your teaching skills or knowledge of medical education; for example, certificates, diplomas or masters in medical education. You may even undertake research in relation to medical education.

You can combine a career in medical education with another in medical academia; however, the two careers are not synonymous. There are potentially four reasons why you may want to be involved in medical education:

- to improve your skills in teaching juniors and students, or to become a student tutor or mentor
- to work in a local postgraduate deanery as a GP tutor, course organiser or clinical tutor
- to become a senior managerial figure in medical education; for example, a senior lecturer in a medical school or postgraduate dean
- to improve the education of medics via research; for example, developing new learning methods like problem-based learning (PBL).

The Association for the Study of Medical Education (ASME) website (www.asme.org.uk) is a good place to gain further information.

References

1 Weissberg P. Research in clinical training. *BMJ Career Focus.* 2002; **325**: 97.

2 Albert T. Publish and prosper. *BMJ Careers.* 1996; **313**: 2.

3 *Modernising Medical Careers Academic Medicine*, 2005. (Available from www.mmc.nhs.uk/pages/careers/academic-medicine)

4 Academic Careers Sub-Committee of *Modernising Medical Careers* and the UK Clinical Research Collaboration. *Medically and Dentally Qualified Staff: recommendations for training the researchers and educators of the future.* Modernising Medical Careers, London, 2005.

Further reading

Academic Medicine Group. *Guidelines for Clinicians Entering Research.* London: RCP; 1997.

British Medical Association. *Medical Academic Career Intentions: results of the BMA cohort study of 1995 medical graduates.* London: BMA; 2004.

British Medical Association. *Role Models in Academic Medicine.* London: BMA; 2005. (Available from www.bma.org.uk)

Research Capacity Development Programme (www.nccrcd.nhs.uk)

Royal College of Physicians. *Clinical Academic Medicine: the way forward.* London: RCP; 2004. (Aimed at those engaged in medical education and research, this report contains clinical academic pathways, with explanations of specific details for each discipline.)

15

GPs with a Special Interest

> The potential roles of GPs are changing; one of these changes is to develop GPs with a 'special interest'. This chapter details how you may become a GP with a Special Interest (GPwSI), the benefits of this and what it involves.

Nearly half of those qualifying as doctors in the UK become GPs. General practice offers opportunities to specialise in a clinical area of interest to you, in addition to the traditional generalist work of a GP. One of the ways in which this occurs is through becoming a GP with a Special Interest (GPwSI).

GPwSIs have developed an additional expertise that expands their clinical practice in a specific field.[1] The rationale and duties of a GPwSI are not the same as GPs who work as hospital practitioners or clinical assistants in hospital or other settings. Nor are they expected to be equivalent to consultants in the corresponding specialty in respect of their caseload. Indeed, GPwSIs work with the support and oversight of hospital consultants in order to provide a wider range of outpatient or community-based services. These may include minor surgery and diagnostic procedures. There is a trend to shift the care of patients from hospital to primary care, and establishing GPwSIs supports this.[2] By having GPwSIs in the locality, patients are able to access services more easily, both more quickly and more conveniently, with more choice in their management. The appointment of a GPwSI should only occur when a review of the local health and service provision of a single primary care trust (PCT), or group of PCTs, is performed and identifies the need.[3]

Subjects in which GPs can develop a special interest include the following.

- The 15 specialties for which the national development group for GPwSI and the Royal College of General Practitioners (RCGP) has produced a set of guidelines and recommendations, which are: care for older people; child protection; coronary heart disease; dermatology; diabetes; drug misuse; echocardiography; emergency care; ear, nose and throat (ENT); epilepsy; headaches; mental health; palliative care; respiratory disease; sexual health (as part of women's and child health).
- Other specialties in which GPs have developed special interests when a need has been identified, include: care of those who find access to traditional health services difficult (e.g. the homeless, asylum seekers, travellers); musculoskeletal medicine; ophthalmology; orthopaedics; procedures suitable for a community setting (endoscopy, cystoscopy, vasectomies).

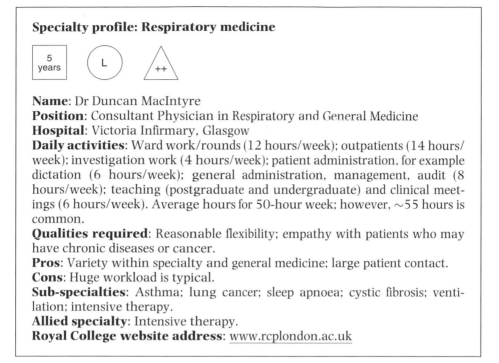

Specialty profile: Respiratory medicine

| 5 years | L | ++ |

Name: Dr Duncan MacIntyre
Position: Consultant Physician in Respiratory and General Medicine
Hospital: Victoria Infirmary, Glasgow
Daily activities: Ward work/rounds (12 hours/week); outpatients (14 hours/week); investigation work (4 hours/week); patient administration, for example dictation (6 hours/week); general administration, management, audit (8 hours/week); teaching (postgraduate and undergraduate) and clinical meetings (6 hours/week). Average hours for 50-hour week; however, ~55 hours is common.
Qualities required: Reasonable flexibility; empathy with patients who may have chronic diseases or cancer.
Pros: Variety within specialty and general medicine; large patient contact.
Cons: Huge workload is typical.
Sub-specialties: Asthma; lung cancer; sleep apnoea; cystic fibrosis; ventilation; intensive therapy.
Allied specialty: Intensive therapy.
Royal College website address: www.rcplondon.ac.uk

As a GPwSI, your priority is to continue as a generalist, but spend about two sessions a week practising your specialty. The benefits to you, as a GPwSI, include lower 'did not attend' (DNA) rates at clinics and structured professional development and education.[2,4] You would be required to set aside up to 15 hours for continuing professional development each year to remain up to date in your specialty field. You should also keep and maintain a portfolio to demonstrate the competencies you have acquired and sustained. Depending on the PCT appointing you, various accreditation schemes are available, including diplomas and local accreditation or certification schemes. A national accreditation group is currently under development by the NHS clinical governance support team (CGST).

References

1 Department of Health. *Practitioners with Special Interests: bringing services close to patients*. London: Department of Health; 2003.

2 Royal College of General Practitioners. *General Practitioners with Special Interests*, 2004. (Available from www.rcgp.org.uk)

3 Department of Health. *Implementing a Scheme for General Practitioners with Special Interests*, 2002. (Available from www.dh.gov.uk/PublicationsAndStatistics/Publications/Publications PolicyAndGuidance/PublicationsPolicyAndGuidanceArticle/fs/en?CONTENT_ID=4009799 &chk=Q3jima)

4 Department of Health. *New Roles for Nurses and GPs to Expand Primary Care and Drive Down Waiting Lists*, 2003. (Available from www.dh.gov.uk/PublicationsAndStatistics/Press Releases/PressReleasesNotices/fs/en?CONTENT_ID=4024519&chk=z8tlp0)

Further reading

Baker M and Chambers R. *A Guide to General Practice Careers*. London: RCGP; 2000.

16

Working abroad

Arranging to work abroad is a complex process. There are many aspects to take into consideration: visas, indemnity, exams, registration, immigration issues, the crime situation – let alone a job to go to and accommodation. This chapter gives you a brief overview of the aspects you should be aware of, or investigate further, before you embark on medical student or postgraduate work or training abroad.

If you have never thought about working abroad before, there are several aspects you should consider.

Think *why* you would want to do so and *what* you would want to get out of the experience. People often decide to work abroad for personal reasons: for a change of pace, maybe to escape from any pressures of home or work, to take unique opportunities, to have greater personal responsibility or just to have some fun. You may want to develop your clinical skills, experience medicine in another culture, go for the teaching, in order to achieve something specific or to stand out from other doctors when it comes to developing your CV.

Think *where* you might want to work; in a developed or less-developed country. If you want to work in third-world countries, especially for voluntary organisations, then they prefer doctors with a reasonable amount of experience rather than relatively junior trainees. There, you are given a lot more responsibility, although conditions may be poor and equipment is often lacking. Do you want to experience Western medicine or maybe traditional Tibetan, Chinese or Outback medicine? If you need to be paid you should go to a developed country.

Think *when* you would like to work abroad. It is widely accepted that the best and most sensible thing to do is to complete the Foundation Programme before doing so. The more junior you are, the less experience you have, but you are also less established in that you are less likely to have a mortgage, children and significant other to keep you in the UK. If you are working overseas later in your career, think about the skills that would be most valuable. For instance, surgical and anaesthetic skills are often extremely useful in third-world countries or in emergency situations such as disaster relief.

Following is information on working in Europe, the United States of America, Australia and Africa. This information is a rough guide to what you should think about if planning to work or train abroad. Each section contains a table, summarising important information about each place.[1] Use the key (Figure 16.1) to interpret these tables. Before you travel you must make sure you research the information provided to make sure it is up to date.

Weather	variable	☼/☁
	hot most of the time	☼
State of healthcare system	poor	✚
	impressive	✚✚✚
Crime		☠
Visas or work permit needed		V
Ease of getting job (easy to very difficult)		☺/☺/☹
Medical needed		♥
Immigration issues		🌍
Exams		✍
Registration		▢
Language tested		Φ
Indemnity insurance required		I
Advance preparation required (months/years)		①②③④/❶❷❸❹
A lot of 'hands-on'		✋
Prevalence of HIV seropositivity		† 26%

Figure 16.1   Icons used to demonstrate working abroad information

Europe

General	☼/☁			
Working	☹	▢ takes 3 months	Φ X not formally tested	♥ X but certificate of good health required

Legislation laid out in 1975, the mutual recognition of medical qualification, resulted in doctors being able to move freely between Austria, Belgium, Denmark, Finland, France, Germany, Greece, Iceland, Ireland, Liechtenstein, Luxemburg, The Netherlands, Norway, Portugal, Spain, Sweden and the UK. You are entitled to full registration in any European Union (EU) country if you are a citizen of a member state and have completed primary training in a member state, obtaining a recognised qualification.

However, as part of the registration process, most authorities or councils require:

- a medical degree certificate
- a certificate of completion of clinical training (CCT) or vocational training (VT) certificate
- passport
- certificate of good standing
- a CV
- a certificate of good health or medical fitness to practise
- evidence of ability to speak the native language.

These may require translation into the country's native language.

United States of America

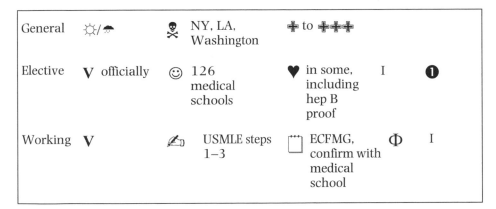

Although three-quarters of the hospitals in the United States of America (USA) are private, the USA is a paradox of excess and deprivation. It is a very popular elective destination, so you are recommended to apply at least a year in advance.

There is a high rate of litigation in the USA, so you must ensure that you have indemnity insurance for your length of stay (*see* Chapter 6). Arranging to work in the USA is a lengthy process, during which time you are required to sit the United States Medical Licensing Examination.

Australia

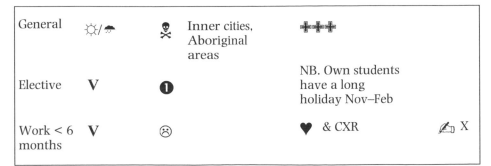

Australia is attractive to many in the UK due to its beautiful sun, sea and surf, no language barrier and being able to practise Western medicine in a relaxed, though still formal, environment. At present Australia has a shortfall in doctors and will have for the next 8–10 years, until the country is able to redress the issue with its own students. Hence, doctors can now earn points for skills towards immigration. Visas are required to work in Australia, but they are complicated. You will have to sit the Australian medical final exams, which contain both undergraduate and postgraduate questions, unless you already have completed specialist training.

Africa

General	☼ Nov–Feb				
Botswana	† 36%	V		☠ X Low crime rate	
The Gambia	† 2%	V if stay > 90 days			
Ghana	† 3.5%				Friendly people, bad roads
Kenya	† 14%	V		☠ recent political turmoil	Φ X but most speak Swahili
Malawi	† 16–30%	V			Girls must NOT show their knees
Namibia	† 20%	V			Basic hygiene problems exist
Nigeria	† 5%	V		Military government	🗒 ✍
South Africa	† 50% in some areas	V		☠ Violence and trauma seen in the townships of Cape Town	✋ Good emergency experience
Tanzania	† 8–20%	V		☠	Most patients speak Swahili

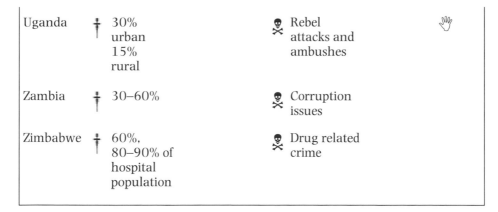

Uganda	30% urban 15% rural	Rebel attacks and ambushes	
Zambia	30–60%	Corruption issues	
Zimbabwe	60%, 80–90% of hospital population	Drug related crime	

Infectious diseases are the biggest medical problem in Africa, for example TB and malaria. In some areas of Africa, HIV seropositivity is as high as 60% (Zimbabwe) so you must be careful when carrying out invasive procedures. Generally, you get a lot of 'hands-on' experience in Africa. However, female doctors must be aware of how they may be viewed in different countries. In Kenya, women may be seen as second-class citizens. In Zimbabwe girls wearing trousers are seen as prostitutes, so you must wear below-the-knee skirts. In Malawi girls must *not* show their legs. You *must* research the area you are planning to visit before you organise your travel, to find out more about their obscure, and more straightforward, customs and traditions.

A final word of advice

In general, plan early. Consider the language, climate, nature and extent of infectious diseases, and state of the healthcare system where you are going, and think of your personal safety. Try to arrange to have a job to come back to before you go. This may involve making an application and succeeding in an interview before you leave.

Reference

1 Wilson M. *The Medic's Guide to Work and Electives around the World*. London: Arnold Publishers; 2000.

17

Diverse medical careers

> You may not have considered all the weird and wonderful career options available to you as a doctor. This chapter will give you a taste of some of the careers you may not have thought of yet.

Working in the defence services

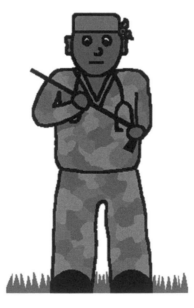

The defence services consist of the Army,[1] Royal Air Force[2] and Royal Navy.[3] Entry can occur from medical student level onwards. The first three years after graduation involves both medical and defence service training. Although differences occur in careers in each military service, this section will give a general idea of what you may expect. It is up to you to get more specific information.

Many disciplines are available in the defence services; from A&E to otorhinolaryng-ology and anaesthetics to ophthalmology.[4] General practice is popular and is the choice of up to 50% of army officers.[5] As in civilian medicine, selection depends upon academic ability and the availability of jobs.

The advantages of working in the defence services are well advertised. Generous bursaries, cadetships and payment of tuition fees are available to medical students. After graduation, the salary compares favourably with that of civilian doctors. Aside from the monetary gains, you can experience the world, gain leadership and management skills, and learn how to cope with the unpredictable.

Disadvantages of a career in the defence services are not so well known, but it is important to consider them carefully. The job is unpredictable: you may be contacted with little or no prior warning to be sent anywhere in the world on service, exercises or on peace keeping and humanitarian operations. You are unlikely to be sent to glamorous places; you can expect to spend time in devastated and dangerous areas. Thus, progress in postgraduate training can be delayed.

Although you are likely to be rich compared with many of your medical school peers, wealth does not come without ties. You will be obligated to serve for at least six years after graduation. Unfortunately, you can never tell how your life may change during medical school, as it is a time when you may go through great personal development. Money may not compensate you for this obligation if your circumstances change.

A survey carried out by the British Medical Association (BMA) of over 200 defence service doctors, covering the three military services, showed that nearly half worked over 50 hours per week. In addition, more than 50% were not able to take their full annual leave entitlement and nearly 10% had spent more than 100 days in deployment on active service over the previous year.[6]

Prison doctor

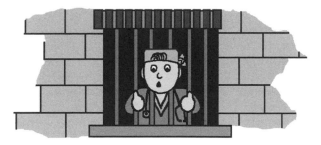

There are a number of openings for GPs to work within the prison medical service, which has only recently become part of the NHS.[7] The Royal Colleges of General Practitioners (RCGP), Physicians (RCP) and Psychiatrists (RCPsych) have designed a diploma in prison medicine. Prison healthcare officers, nurses and pharmacists will support your work. In addition, visiting specialists, such as psychiatrists, dentists and optometrists, may hold clinics in prisons.[8]

As patients, the majority of inmates are needy. Many come from deprived backgrounds and they are often homeless. Therefore, other than routine medical screening of new inmates and GP work, a prison doctor's caseload often involves the management of problems common to many prisoners: mental health problems, substance misuse and communicable diseases. In addition, as their advocate you should ensure that the conditions of detention are not having a deleterious effect on their health – either mental or physical. Drawbacks of this career include possible demands by prison staff and authorities that could conflict with your ethical obligations. It is important you are aware of this so that you can manage such situations appropriately.

Ship's doctor

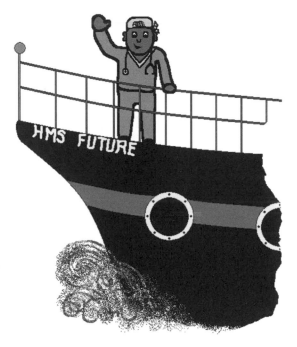

Does sailing the seas while trying to save lives (!) appeal to you? Being a ship's doctor,[9] you will have the opportunity to experience more of the world and its people. Being able to communicate well and being sociable are essential.

If you choose to work on a cruise liner you can expect very well-equipped facilities. Many such vessels have onboard X-ray facilities, an intensive therapy unit (ITU), mini-laboratory for testing blood, pharmacy, a treatment room that doubles up as an operating theatre and several wards for inpatients.

Contracts may be four to eight months in length. Depending on the size of the ship, and the number of doctors, you will be expected to run one or two clinics a day. All patients are seen on a private basis, therefore some will be more demanding and will require a more tolerant attitude. If uniforms do not 'float your boat' you need to think of another career. Expect to wear an officer's uniform whenever you are near passenger areas.

The most essential training experience you would need is in general practice. You should also have had rotations in A&E and had experience on ITU. For some jobs you are required to have at least three years' experience in emergency medicine. Other useful areas to experience during your training would be general medicine, care of the elderly and psychiatry. In addition, you must also have gained an advanced cardiac life support certificate. If you are planning on being a doctor on a ship with American passengers you will also be required to complete the advanced trauma life support course.

Media doctor

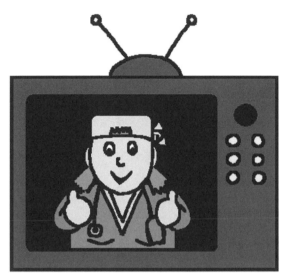

Being a media doctor may be the career for you if you enjoy explaining things clearly. You can be a media doctor in various ways: writing (including technical work), radio, television and the internet. It can be fun and a chance to communicate with many people.

However, becoming a media doctor is not easy, and being successful is even harder. Initially, many write for papers and magazines. You can move on from writing comments, to features, articles, health columns or even books. Getting on radio and television is even more difficult. There are few openings and, as anything can be thrown at you, you require training in both medical and media skills. You also need to be engaging, something which may not come naturally to you.[10]

As a media doctor, you cannot guarantee when each job will arise and you can expect to get limited time for preparation. However, it is possible to practise part-time medicine whilst being in the media, to provide some stability.

Not everyone will agree with what you do. As a media doctor, not only are you leaving yourself open for misrepresentation, you are exposing yourself to potential hostility from patients, the public and even your colleagues.[11]

Medicine and the law

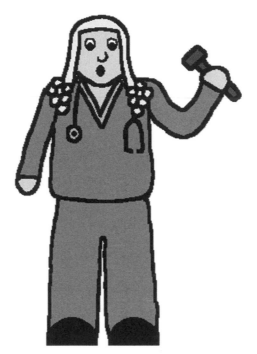

Only a few careers accommodate both medicine and law:[12] being a coroner and regulatory work within the pharmaceutical industry. However, if you are already a doctor but would like to work in a legal-related field there are a number of options, including forensic pathology, forensic psychiatry, police surgeon, prison doctor, medical adviser for a medical defence organisation or court or other legal professions and academics in forensic medicine, forensic sciences or medical law and ethics.

Generally, once you have completed two years as a specialist registrar, you can concentrate on one of the specialties mentioned above. It is possible to obtain a diploma in forensic medicine or law. However, as a doctor you are unlikely to get financial support to study for a legal qualification.

Skills required include the ability to explain technical information in a concise manner, which is understandable to lay people. You should also have the confidence to handle widely publicised cases and to withstand harsh cross-examination in court.

Premier league doctor

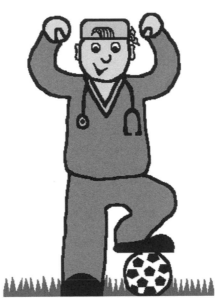

You want football to be your life and being a doctor will be your life, so why not combine the two? It is not difficult to see the drawbacks of wanting to be a premier league doctor,[13,14] not least the number of premier league teams there are across the country. Therefore, setting your sights on sports medicine in local teams may be best initially. The principle is the same and, who knows, you might get lucky.

GP training is the usual starting block, followed by a diploma in sports medicine. Rotations during training should include general medicine and A&E. Other useful placements would be rheumatology and orthopaedics. Once trained, GPs are expected to spend at least half their time dedicated to sports and exercise medicine to be deemed competent. As a premier league doctor you would be spending 100% of your time working in sports medicine.

Good experience can be gained by working and volunteering with local teams; however, you must have appropriate training otherwise you will not be protected against litigation.

Life as a premier league doctor is not all glamorous. You would be on call around the clock and have to travel everywhere that the team goes. If musculoskeletal examination is not your forte you would have to work hard to change this or think again. Currently, sports medicine is not recognised by the royal colleges as a specialty in its own right. However, several UK universities offer diplomas in sports medicines.

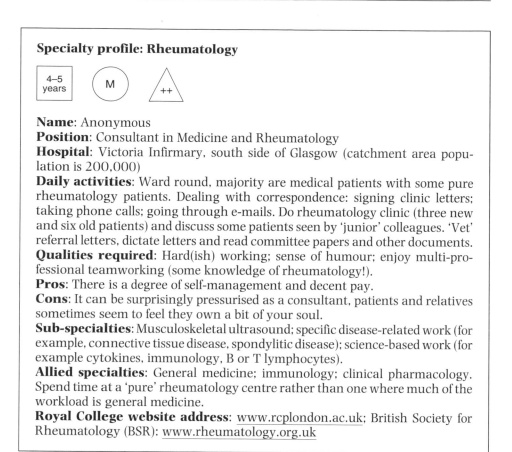

Specialty profile: Rheumatology

4–5 years | M | ++

Name: Anonymous

Position: Consultant in Medicine and Rheumatology

Hospital: Victoria Infirmary, south side of Glasgow (catchment area population is 200,000)

Daily activities: Ward round, majority are medical patients with some pure rheumatology patients. Dealing with correspondence: signing clinic letters; taking phone calls; going through e-mails. Do rheumatology clinic (three new and six old patients) and discuss some patients seen by 'junior' colleagues. 'Vet' referral letters, dictate letters and read committee papers and other documents.

Qualities required: Hard(ish) working; sense of humour; enjoy multi-professional teamworking (some knowledge of rheumatology!).

Pros: There is a degree of self-management and decent pay.

Cons: It can be surprisingly pressurised as a consultant, patients and relatives sometimes seem to feel they own a bit of your soul.

Sub-specialties: Musculoskeletal ultrasound; specific disease-related work (for example, connective tissue disease, spondylitic disease); science-based work (for example cytokines, immunology, B or T lymphocytes).

Allied specialties: General medicine; immunology; clinical pharmacology. Spend time at a 'pure' rheumatology centre rather than one where much of the workload is general medicine.

Royal College website address: www.rcplondon.ac.uk; British Society for Rheumatology (BSR): www.rheumatology.org.uk

References

1   Royal Army Medical Corps. *What Does Army Medicine Involve?* (Available from www. army.mod.uk/medical/royal_army_medical_corps/careers_in_the_ramc/medical_officer_ doctor/what_does_army_medicine_involve/index.htm)

2   Royal Air Force Careers. *Medical Officers.* (Available from www.rafcareers.com/jobs/ job_files/jobfile_medicalofficer.cfm)

3   Royal Navy. *Medical Officer.* (Available from www.royal-navy.mod.uk/static/pages/ 3355.html)

4   Royal Army Medical Corps. *Hospital Specialisation.* (Available from www.army.mod.uk/ medical/royal_army_medical_corps/careers_in_the_ramc/medical_officer_doctor/ hospital_specialist/index.htm)

5   Royal Army Medical Corps. *General Practice.* (Available from www.army.mod.uk/medical/ royal_army_medical_corps/careers_in_the_ramc/medical_officer_doctor/gp/index.htm)

6   British Medical Association. *Armed Forces Doctors' Pay Rise Fails to Address Recruitment and Retention Crisis.* 26 May 2005. (Available from www.bma.org.uk)

7   Aquino P and Jones P. *Career Options in General Practice.* Oxford: Radcliffe Publishing; 2004.

8   Longfield M. Opportunities for doctors in the prison service. *BMJ Career Focus*. 1999; **318**: 2.

9   Shafi S. Working as a ship's doctor. *BMJ Career Focus*. 1998; **316**: 2.

10   Easton G. Working in the media 1: options for doctors. *StudentBMJ*. 2004; **12**: 194–6.

11   Stillman P. Developing skills for the broadcast media. *BMJ Careers*. 1997; **314**: 2.

12   Leung WC. Career focus: combining medicine and law. *StudentBMJ*. 2000; **8**: 68–9.

13   Welch W and Kelly S. Premier league doctor. *StudentBMJ*. 2004; **12**: 286.

14   English B. Sports and exercise medicine. *StudentBMJ*. 2004; **12**: 282–3.

Further reading

Defence Deanery (www.gprecruitment.org.uk/deanery/defence/index.htm)

Defence Medical Services Department (www.dsmd.mod.uk)

Easton G. Working in the media 2: getting a foot in the door. *StudentBMJ*. 2004; **12**: 240–1.

Easton G. Working in the media 3: getting your message across. *StudentBMJ*. 2004; **12**: 284–5.

Kenny F. Creative medicine. *StudentBMJ*. 2006; **14**: 104–5.

www.bma.org.uk/ap.nsf/Content/Hubarmedforcesdoctors. (Section of the BMA website on working in the armed forces.)

Beasley R, Aldington S and Robinson G. From medical student to junior doctor: working outside the box. *StudentBMJ*. 2006; **14**: 238–9.

Sritharan K. A life on the ocean wave. *StudentBMJ*. 2006; **14**: 244–5.

18

What else can I do with a degree in medicine?

This chapter is designed to give advice and make you aware of the options available to you should you decide that medicine is not for you.

Although most medical students can deal with the demands of an intensive course, some may find the pressure too intense. In every medical school there should be someone you can talk to about any problems you are having on your course. For instance there may be a mentoring scheme in your medical school. More information on this can be found in Chapter 5. Those students who, in the first two years, feel that they no longer want to continue with medicine can sometimes transfer to another related course, such as pharmacology or biomedical sciences. Students who have managed to progress through the first year of clinical training may then decide that they do not want to continue studying medicine and those who fail finals and re-sits may be eligible to be awarded a degree of biomedical science.

Even some medical students who manage to graduate choose not to work in medicine and may opt to pursue an alternative career. The knowledge that they gained whilst studying medicine may be invaluable in their new career. Careers related to medicine include medical journalism, medico-legal practice or working for the pharmaceutical industry. However, employers may prefer to appoint someone who has progressed further in their career and who has gained clinical experience by practising medicine. So if these careers do interest you it might be useful to stay in the NHS for a few years after qualifying to improve your chances in your chosen career outside mainstream medicine.

Medical graduates who go into careers that do not involve medicine are at a disadvantage compared with those who do. This is because they are only using their degree as currency, rather than as an advantage to their chosen career. They may take a drop in salary as they change professions and may have decreased job security. Their pension rights may also be compromised.

The decision not to practise medicine or work in the medical field is hard. It should not be done for financial reasons, as you can end up earning less money, having lower job security and poorer pension structures by leaving the NHS. If you think that you cannot deal with the demands placed on you by your medical career you should first step back and stop yourself from making a rash decision. There are ways of dealing with this pressure, for example:

- seeking career guidance
- adjusting your working conditions, for example flexible working

- addressing and amending, as appropriate, your work–life balance.

Alternatively, if you decide to take a break from medicine there may be incentive schemes to help you to return to the NHS at a later date. For example, the flexible returner scheme, which is part of the Flexible Careers Scheme, may still be available to you (*see* Chapter 12).

If you are considering leaving medical school or the medical profession, first take a look at chapters 11 and 12. They might just make you change your mind!

Further reading

Adams J. Is there life after medicine? *BMJ Career Focus*. 2003; **327**: 86.

Chambers R, Mohanna K and Field S. *Opportunities and Options in Medical Careers*. Oxford: Radcliffe Medical Press; 2000.

19

Societies and organisations

This chapter introduces you to some of the societies and organisations that you may be in contact with throughout your medical career. The information has been written and/or approved by the organisations involved, which accounts for the slight variation in style and consistency of the writing; however, it ensures that information was correct at the time of print.

General Medical Council

Main roles: accountability, discipline, registration, advice

The General Medical Council (GMC) has the legal power to protect, promote and maintain the health and safety of the community by ensuring proper standards in the practice of medicine.

The responsibilities of the GMC are listed below.

- Co-ordinates all stages and promotes high standards in medical association.
- Provisionally registers graduates of UK medical schools.
- Publishes guidance on general clinical training and its implementation.
- Grants full registration to doctors who gain the required competencies.
- Maintains a list and publishes a register of specialist doctors and, in the future, a list of GPs.
- Recognises qualifications awarded by EEA member states to EEA nationals.
- Regulates doctors.

The GMC website contains the guidelines mentioned above. These guidelines are useful and important in your education and practice throughout medical school. Other areas covered by the guidelines include consent of patients and conduct as a health professional (and medical student).

Website (www.gmc-uk.org)

Postgraduate Medical Education and Training Board

Main roles: postgraduate medical education and training

The Postgraduate Medical Education and Training Board (PMETB) is an independent statutory body, responsible for overseeing and promoting the development of post-graduate medical education and training for all specialties, including general practice, across the UK.

It assumed its statutory powers on 30 September 2005, taking over the responsibilities of the Specialist Training Authority (STA) of the medical royal colleges and the Joint Committee on Postgraduate Training for General Practice (JCPTGP).

The vision that PMETB has set itself is to achieve excellence in postgraduate medical education, training, assessment and accreditation throughout the UK to improve the knowledge, skills and experience of doctors and the health and healthcare of patients and the public.

The General and Specialist Medical Practice (Education, Training and Qualifications) Order 2003 (Statutory Instrument 2003 No. 1250) established the PMETB and defines its purpose – to regulate and develop postgraduate medical education and training.

Under the Order, the PMETB is responsible for:

- establishing standards and requirements for postgraduate medical education and training
- making sure these standards and requirements are met
- developing and promoting postgraduate medical education and training across the country.

The statutory objectives of the PMETB are to:

- safeguard the health and well-being of persons using the services of GPs or specialists
- ensure that the needs of persons undertaking postgraduate medical education and training in each of the countries of the United Kingdom are met by the standards it establishes
- ensure that the needs of employers and those engaging the services of GPs and specialists within the NHS are met.

Website (www.pmetb.org.uk)

British Medical Association

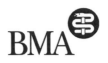

Main roles: advice, protection (of rights)

The British Medical Association (BMA) is the professional association for all UK doctors, and an independent trade union that is recognised by the government as a scientific and educational body, with sole negotiating rights for doctors. As such, it represents doctors from all branches of medicine all over the UK, and has over 135,000 members, including over 16,000 student members.

The main aims of the BMA are to protect and support its members' professional interests and to negotiate with the government and NHS Employers to bring about improvements in the profession and the NHS.

Student members receive a monthly copy of *StudentBMJ*, containing interesting political, lifestyle and educational articles, and opinions of medical students, accompanied by *Student BMA News*, featuring news, views and analysis.

For full details on the benefits of membership, visit the BMA website.

Website (www.bma.org.uk/join)

Medical Defence Union

Main roles: advice, protection

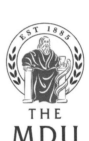

The Medical Defence Union (MDU) is a mutual, non-profit organisation, owned by its members – doctors, dentists and other healthcare professionals. Established in 1885, the MDU was the first medical defence organisation in the UK and provides members with advice and support throughout their studies and professional lives.

As well as providing all the traditional discretionary benefits of a mutual, the MDU also provides its qualified members with the security of an insurance policy for indemnity up to £10 million.*

Other benefits of membership include:

* indemnity for Good Samaritan acts performed worldwide*
* access to Freephone 24-hour advisory helpline
* discounted books, courses and educational services
* defence of professional reputations if clinical performance is called into question
* support in responding to patient complaints
* support with GMC or NHS disciplinary proceedings
* access to the MDU press office assisting with enquiries from the media
* access to case histories and advisory publications within the MDU website.

For further information about the benefits of MDU membership visit the website (www.the-mdu.com) or contact the Membership Helpline on 0800 716376.

Website (www.the-mdu.com)

*Subject to the terms and conditions of the Professional Indemnity Policy underwritten by Converium Insurance (UK) Ltd.

MDU Services Limited (MDUSL) is authorised and regulated by the Financial Services Authority in respect of insurance mediation activities only. MDUSL is an agent for The Medical Defence Union Limited (the MDU). The MDU is not an insurance company. The benefits of membership of the MDU are all discretionary and are subject to the Memorandum and Articles of Association.

MDU Services Limited is registered in England 3957086 Registered Office: 230 Blackfriars Road London SE1 8PJ.

Medical and Dental Defence Union of Scotland

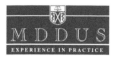

Main roles: advice, protection, risk management

The Medical and Dental Defence Union of Scotland (MDDUS) is an independent UK-wide mutual indemnity organisation providing members with comprehensive indemnity and 24-hour advice and support.

Currently, the MDDUS has 25,000 members and is managed and governed by medical and dental practitioners. The aims of the MDDUS are to protect the professional interests of its members and to promote high standards of medical and dental practice.

Members have 24/7 access to clinically qualified medical advisers, uniquely experienced professionals with extensive understanding of the variety of situations encountered. This enables all situations to be managed sympathetically, effectively and in strict confidence.

Other services provided for members include:

- occurrence-based indemnity and support for legal action brought about by patients against general medical practitioners and specialists in private practice
- assistance with complaints
- professional advice and legal representation at GMC proceedings
- legal representation at fatal accident inquiries and coroner's inquests
- indemnity for assisting at emergencies and other occasions such as voluntary hospice work and worldwide Good Samaritan acts
- representation at disciplinary proceedings
- quarterly publication, *Summons*
- access to risk management advice in general medical practice
- advice and indemnity for the preparation of reports and expert opinions
- continued indemnity, after the member has ceased clinical practice, or left membership, for the period that they were in membership
- the option to put membership on hold if not working due to retirement, maternity leave or ill health – indemnity for Good Samaritan acts and *Summons* are still provided free of charge.

Membership costs depend upon specialty and length of practice, for advice on this you can contact the MDDUS. However, free membership is available to medical and dental students throughout the UK. Student membership provides benefits, including:

- a leather diary
- free advice booklets on topical medico-legal and practice issues
- quarterly publication, *Summons*, includes case studies and student pages
- discount on clinical textbooks from specified publishers, see the MDDUS website for further details
- involvement and sponsorship of student events, see the MDDUS website for further details.

Website (www.mddus.com)

Medical Protection Society

MEDICAL PROTECTION SOCIETY

Main roles: advice, protection

The Medical Protection Society (MPS) prides itself on being the world's leading mutual medical protection organisation. It has the aim of providing help, in the form of protection and advice, to healthcare professionals with medico-legal problems that arise from their clinical practice.

A 24-hour telephone emergency advice line is offered. Services provided by the MPS are confidential. Specific and general situations that MPS members can ask for assistance with include:

- clinical negligence claims
- complaints
- legal and ethical dilemmas
- GMC inquiries
- disciplinary procedures
- inquests and fatal accident inquiries
- police investigations relating to clinical practice.

In addition to assisting healthcare professionals with the above situations, the MPS also:

- has a role in risk management – working to promote safer practice
- lobbies to bring about a sensible regulatory environment
- can provide indemnity
- can provide legal representation
- can act as a spokesperson to the media.

The assistance offered by the MPS is given at the discretion of the MPS council, which consists mainly of medical and dental practitioners.

The MPS publishes a really useful journal, *Casebook*, as part of its work in promoting patient safety. *Casebook* is sent out to all MPS members and contains educational articles, letters and a really useful section that details previous cases where legal action has been sought. This latter section details the history of the case and what the outcome was. It then goes on to explain where errors occurred or what was good about the management. It is a really interesting tool that draws your attention to errors that have easily been made, but are potentially easy to avoid.

Website (www.mps.org.uk)

Howden Medical Insurance Services   Howden >

Main roles: advice, protection

Complaints and allegations of negligence or poor performance against medical practitioners are undoubtedly on the rise. On average a dentist or doctor is expected to receive one formal complaint for every two years they are in practice. Howden Medical Insurance Services (HMIS) is a new commercial company. However, the professional and medical risks division of Howden Insurance Brokers prides itself in having longstanding expertise in the field of medical malpractice. Doctors and dentists need to know that they have an indemnity insurance that is secure, reliable and supported by fully trained and experienced medico-legal experts. Backed by a consortium of London insurers, the HMIS team of medical, dental and claims specialists has launched a service tailored to meet the individual needs of dentists and doctors. HMIS provides cover for groups or individuals including: health authorities, medical associations, medical training colleges/universities, hospitals (public and private sector), clinics, medical practitioners (doctors, dentists, surgeons, chiropractors, osteopaths), other medical professionals (opticians, paramedics, pharmacists, nurses, chiropodists) and complementary medical practitioners (acupuncturists, homeopaths).

The cover HMIS offers may include:

- public and products liability
- protection against libel and slander
- cover for loss of documents.
- supplementary legal expenses cover
- access to a range of helplines
- a range of 'run off' options.

Website (www.hmis.co.uk)

Wesleyan Medical Sickness

Main roles: financial advice, income protection

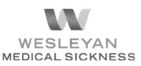

Have you ever thought about what you would do if accident or illness prevented you from working and earning an income? The Medical Career Protector from Wesleyan Assurance Society is specifically designed for medical students and doctors. Exclusively provided through Wesleyan Medical Sickness, it is designed to protect your income should you suffer loss of earnings as a result of illness or accident. As a final-year medical student they can arrange cover for you free of charge, as they understand it is cover that you may not be able to afford. Then when you qualify as a doctor, just £24 per month will help to provide the cover you'll need in the early years of your career. In 2004 the Society paid over £36 million pounds in claims to doctors and dentists who were unable to work.

Wesleyan Medical Sickness has a dedicated team of Student Liaison Managers covering medical schools across the UK who can provide information about and access to the cover. In addition they can provide sponsorship to school clubs, societies and events such as your Graduation Ball. They will also be co-ordinating your group photo – a tradition that Wesleyan Medical Sickness has upheld for over 30 years. Medical Sickness gives this photo to each and every final-year student, as a free gift from them, to remind you of your years at medical school.

Wesleyan Medical Sickness has been addressing the needs of medics since 1884 and is part of the Wesleyan Assurance Society, one of the oldest and financially strong mutual organisations in the UK. They also offer a wide range of insurance products for students, covering elective travel, motor and personal possessions.

Website (www.wesleyanmedicalsickness.co.uk)

Medical Women's Federation

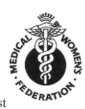

Main roles: advice, representation of women in medicine

The Medical Women's Federation (MWF) is the largest and most influential body of women doctors in the UK.

The aims are to support women doctors in their personal and professional development, to remove gender barriers in the medical profession at all levels, and to improve the health of women and their families in society.

Annual student sponsorship:

- annual essay competition open to all medical students
- grants for medical student electives
- mature student grants for those with financial hardship.

They campaign on a number of issues, including flexible working and childcare, have representation on all important medical committees, input into major health policies and documents and, as part of the Medical Women's International Association, look at women's health issues globally.

Website (www.medicalwomensfederation.org.uk)

PasTest

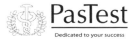

Main roles: education, career support

With over 30 years' experience of helping doctors and medical students pass their exams, PasTest provides high quality medical education. It provides a combination of books, courses, online revision, continuing professional development conferences and exhibitions. PasTest offers a complete career solution to medical students and doctors of all disciplines.

Website (www.pastest.co.uk)

20

Discrimination and how to avoid it

> Discrimination is unacceptable. However, it is a real phenomenon occurring in medicine, as in other professions. It may not be apparent to everyone which groups or individuals are more vulnerable to discrimination or how this discrimination is manifested. This chapter highlights these points and suggests ways to avoid discrimination and, if it is already occurring, from where help can be sought.

Discrimination can occur as a result of illness, disease, disability, disfigurement, education, ethnic origin, religion, gender, age and sexual orientation. This list is not exhaustive, but it illustrates the diversity of traits that can lead to discrimination, and thus that discrimination could occur towards any of us. Discrimination may not be overt; all of us must be aware that we could each be a victim of discrimination. It is best to attempt to prevent discrimination from occurring in the first place as many people are reluctant to act against discrimination once it occurs, for fear of creating a detrimental effect on their career.

Negative effects of discrimination can include unhappiness, isolation and low self-esteem. In terms of careers, discrimination may result in limited and difficult career progression.

A career in medicine involves interaction with all members of the community from all walks of life. It is important that you understand how and why discrimination develops and is manifested so you will recognise it if you start to become a perpetrator.

Discrimination, or more accurately, preventing discrimination, is a major theme of General Medical Council (GMC), Royal College and National Health Service (NHS) legislation and guidelines. The GMC *Good Medical Practice*, *Tomorrow's Doctors* and *Duties of a Doctor* publications (*see* Chapter 9) each promote fair treatment of patients and colleagues. The NHS has set up flexible working, childcare, training and work-force retention initiatives to open up the opportunities of work to more people.[1] The British Medical Association has insisted that bullying must stop and thus recommends zero tolerance. They have produced the report, *Bullying and Harassment of Doctors in the Workplace*, which can be found at www.bma.org.uk/ap.nsf/Content/bullying2006.

Forms of discrimination

There are five basic types of discrimination.

Direct discrimination

Discrimination occurring directly as a result of a trait of a person (e.g. age, disability, religion, race, sex or sexual orientation). This discrimination would not occur should this trait not be present. Complainants alleging direct discrimination have to compare themselves with either an actual or hypothetical comparator to illustrate less-favourable treatment.

Indirect discrimination

This occurs when a provision/criterion/practice is applied equally to all people but the effect of this is detrimental to a group of people because a considerably smaller proportion of people sharing a particular characteristic are able to comply.

Victimisation

Victimisation is unlawfully present when one person treats another less favourably than they treat others because the person has brought proceedings under a relevant piece of discrimination legislation, given evidence or information in connection with proceedings under a relevant piece of discrimination legislation, alleged that someone has contravened a relevant piece of discrimination legislation, or because the person believes that the victim has done or intends to do these things.

Harassment

This is said to occur when one person engages in unwanted conduct with another, based on a specific trait (e.g. sex, race, disability, etc.), which may violate that person's dignity or create an unpleasant environment for that person, for example intimidation, humiliation, offence.

Bullying

This is said to occur when power or status is misused to criticise, condemn and humiliate people, which may result in undermining their ability and/or confidence.

Gender issues

Gender is a dynamic cause of discrimination. Not only are proportions of men and women in medicine changing, but various specialties have differing male/female preponderances. Between 1990 and 2000, the total number of female hospital medical staff increased by 71%. In addition, the number of women entering medical school has doubled since the 1980s, with less than a 10% increase in male entrants over the same time.[2]

   You may look at these figures and assume that women now dominate medicine, and that previous gender-based discrimination may be a thing of the past. However, women's progression in hospital medicine has been slower than expected and in 1998 only 20% of hospital consultants were women.[2]

Surgery has particularly low ratios of female to male consultants and registrars. Conversely, the greatest female to male ratios occur in clinical oncology, paediatrics, pathology, psychiatry and obstetrics and gynaecology.[2,3]

So what can be done with this information? First, do not let it put you off going into a specialty you are interested in. Discrimination can be so diverse that even if you are in a minority group it may not occur towards you if you are a female going into surgery. For instance, a 'Women in Surgical Training' initiative was established to encourage this by the Royal College of Surgeons and the Department of Health. Whether the apparent gender bias in various specialties is really due to discrimination or lifestyle choice is unclear. Be aware and ensure your chosen career path is not obscured by discrimination.

Transgender doctors may also present the potential for discrimination. Although many are happy and comfortable with their own situation, some may not be open about their sexuality for fear of others' negative reactions.

Sexual orientation

Many gay, lesbian and bisexual people are comfortable with their sexuality; however, fear of negative reactions from colleagues or patients can result in them not opening up to such people.[4] MacDonald stated that only half of clinical students believe homosexual activity can form part of an acceptable lifestyle.[5]

As a rule, when doctors are open about their sexuality, they have no problem. Discrimination in employment on the basis of sexual orientation is illegal – however, the possibility remains.[4]

Ethnic origin

Ethnic minorities make up a significant proportion of medical professionals. Around one-third of hospital doctors are non-white.[2] However, these figures do not represent the situation at more senior levels: 80% of consultants and 64% of registrars are white. Even at senior house officer (SHO) level over half of all doctors are white. How much of this bias is due to discrimination may remain unclear, but if you are from a minority ethnic group, you should be vigilant as to meeting unfair or discriminatory treatment.

Illness, disease and disability

Physical and mental illness can result in discrimination. In a world of 'caring professionals' the same professionals do not always appear as such when their own colleagues, or medical students, are involved. In particular, mental illness is a significant cause of discrimination.[5]

If you are disabled, your employers must not treat you less favourably as a result of your disability, unless action is justified. They must make reasonable adjustments to your working conditions or workplace to enable you to work more effectively/easily. If your employer does not comply with these requirements they may be discriminating against you and you should research your rights, starting with the Disability

Discrimination Act 1995 (DDA). It is important to realise the extent of the DDA. It covers disability caused by a wide range of conditions, for example cancer, HIV and facial disfigurement.

How to avoid discriminating against patients and colleagues

- Identify your own prejudices. We all have them and it is only by identifying them that we can attempt to prevent them from affecting our professional work and judgement.
- Remember that medical students and doctors with disabilities have already illustrated determination, intellectual ability and skills to get where they are – do not write them off.
- Understand your personality type (*see* Chapter 3) – the Myers–Briggs Type Indicator, a psychometric test used worldwide, involves a dimension which focuses on the way in which people make decisions. Grouping people by their decision-making styles, into 'thinkers' and 'feelers', creates groups, which may explain the development of bullying and/or discrimination. Thinkers are said to be exhilarated by conflict and may appear as tactless or abusive to feelers, despite the thinkers' intention being quite different. By understanding whether you are a thinker or a feeler, you may be able to manage situations which may result in an act of discrimination more appropriately.[6]
- Read articles about, or listen to, other people's experiences of discrimination and learn from them.
- Be aware of and avoid stereotyping people.
- Assess an individual's competencies and abilities based on their own merits.
- Be aware that it is illegal to discriminate against people at work on the grounds of sex, sexual orientation, race, religion, disability, part-time working or being, or not being, a member of a trades union.
- Realise that people with chronic conditions are often the experts of their own medical problems and lifestyle requirements; if you are unsure of anything just ask.

How to avoid being discriminated against

Giving generic tips on how to avoid discrimination directed at you is difficult due to the diversity of traits that result in discrimination. The following list has been written to be interpreted in a 'where applicable' fashion.

- Be open and honest with yourself and your colleagues,[7] you do not have to tell everyone in every case, but make sure you are honest with those to whom it legally and ethically matters.
- Maintain your health at the best that you can while avoiding excessive time off work – time off work can lead to time out of training and thus a deficiency of skills or knowledge:
  - try and keep doctors' appointments out of your working hours if possible
  - be compliant with your medication and treatment

- generally maintain good health by eating regularly and taking regular breaks, especially if you need more than others due to illness.
- Identify problems you have which may lead to discrimination and think about ways of overcoming or adapting to these problems[7] – this may include the use of aids, gadgets or alterations to the workplace.
- Seek help from relevant people or organisations, which may include:
  - colleagues
  - employers – they are liable for acts of discrimination carried out by their employees, regardless of knowledge or approval; employers are also liable if considered to have failed to have prevented employees suffering discrimination in the workplace, where possible, therefore, it is in your employer's interest to take a part in preventing discrimination
  - postgraduate deanery
  - occupational health department
  - support groups – limited details can be found in Appendix 1
  - 'Access to Work' – a government scheme run through local job centre plus offices which conducts workplace assessments and can provide advice on and funding for (in certain circumstances) extra equipment or costs incurred which may be needed for your employment
  - *BMJ Careers* chronic illness matching scheme
  - Association for Disabled Professionals – provides advice and runs a network support scheme which matches professionals with similar disabilities and jobs to provide support for each other
  - Workstep – will put you in touch with a disability employment adviser and provides job support to disabled employees
  - Disability Rights Commission (DRC), Commission for Racial Equality (CRE) and Equal Opportunities Commission (EOC) – provide advice, support and legal information to help you ensure the rights of the groups they represent are protected.
- Know your rights and do not be forced into decisions you will regret (e.g. lower posts, retirement) – certain documents, acts and regulations have been produced and organisations exist to assist with legal issues:
  - The Disability Discrimination Act 1995 – produced to ensure employers fulfil their responsibilities to you and provide additional resources to assist you in performing your job[7]
  - Sex Discrimination Act 1975 – it is illegal to discriminate against people at work on the basis of sex
  - The Employment Equality (sexual orientation) Regulations 2003 – it is illegal to discriminate against people at work on the basis of their sexual orientation
  - Race Relations Act 1976 – covers discrimination on the grounds of race
  - The Employment Equality (religion or belief) Regulations 2003 – covers discrimination on the grounds of religion
  - Prevention of Less Favourable Treatment Regulations 2000 – produced to prevent discrimination of part-time workers, ensuring equal pay, inclusion in appropriate training, adequate holiday entitlement, availability of career break schemes (e.g. maternity leave) and fair consideration at times of redundancy
  - Disability Rights Commission (DRC), Commission for Racial Equality (CRE) and Equal Opportunities Commission (EOC) (*see above*).

Lastly, it is important that you ensure you maintain good social relationships to provide a good source of support should these preventative measures fail.

What you can do if discrimination occurs

Your instinct may be not to act. However, you should think carefully before doing this. If you feel you are being discriminated against, the chances are some of your colleagues may be as well. This decision should be made relatively quickly, as you only have three months minus one day from the date of the act of discrimination to submit an application to an employment tribunal.[1]

If you make a complaint of discrimination your employer is expected to deal with this promptly, objectively, thoroughly and with due regard to confidentiality. They are duty bound to do this, not only for your benefit but for their own. The employer's commitment to equal opportunities will be judged on the basis of how they deal with situations such as this. If your employer does not deal with your complaint appropriately their actions may be interpreted as approval of the discrimination.[1]

In order to make a good case for discrimination, bullying or harassment you will need to collect evidence and record details of what has been happening. Keeping a diary, which logs the events and any witnesses, can be helpful. In addition, any letters, e-mails or other permanent items of communication should be kept.[8]

The British Medical Association (BMA) will take on cases of members only if their associated lawyers decide they have at least a 50% chance of winning. For those whose cases are not taken on, the BMA also offers their members a counselling line for support.[9]

Once you have taken action for alleged discrimination, the case will be assessed for its suitability to be resolved informally. However, it is also recommended that you submit an application to an employment tribunal immediately due to tight time restrictions. If your case is not deemed suitable for informal resolution it will be passed through your employer's procedure for dealing with complaints of alleged discrimination. Severe cases may require resolution under your employer's disciplinary policy.[1]

References

1 British Medical Association. *Dealing with Discrimination: guidelines for BMA members.* London: BMA; 2004.

2 Jackson C, Ball JE, Hirsh W et al. *Informing Choices: the need for career advice in medical training.* Cambridge: National Institute for Careers Education Counselling; 2003.

3 Allen I. Women doctors and their careers: what now. *BMJ.* 2005; **331**: 569–72.

4 Gay and Lesbian Association of Doctors and Dentists, 2005. (Available from www. gladd.dircon.co.uk)

5 MacDonald R. Discrimination in medicine. *BMJ.* 2002; **324**: 1112.

6 Paice E and Firth-Cozens J. Who's a bully then. *BMJ Career Focus.* 2003; **326**: 127.

7 Stiff RE. Life as a visually impaired doctor. *BMJ Career Focus.* 2004; **329**: 15–16.

8 British Medical Association Career Focus. *Overseas Doctors: sink or swim.* London: BMA; 2004.

9 Cohen D and Hebert K. Equality and diversity in the workplace. *BMJ Career Focus*. 2004; **329**: 116–17.

Further reading

British Medical Association. *Sexual Orientation in the Workplace*. London: BMA; 2005.

Gay and Lesbian Association of Doctors and Dentists. *Improving Working Lives: guidelines on dignity at work for lesbian and gay doctors and dentists, medical and dental students*, 2004. (Available from www.gladd.org.uk)

Appendix 1

Resources

Chapter 1: Introduction

- BMJ Careers (www.bmjcareers.com). There is a 'users guide' leaflet to accompany this.
- Modernising Medical Careers (www.mmc.nhs.uk). Look specifically at the frequently asked questions page on Foundation training. Also from here you can find links to all deanery websites which provide the following information: facilities, career advice, training offered, process of application, closing dates of application.

Chapter 2: Experiences of others

- Doctors.net (www.doctors.net).
- GP recruitment (www.gprecruitment.org.uk). Includes information on GP careers, day in the life of a GP, qualities of a good GP, vacancies, information and links to all UK deanery websites.

Chapter 3: Career development toolkit

- Competition ratios (www.bmjcareers.com/cgi-bin/section.pl?sn=juniorcomp). Contains information on competition for jobs at PRHO/F1 and SHO/F2 level and also information about different areas of the country.
- *The Lancet* (www.thelancet.com).
- London Deanery (www.londondeanery.ac.uk).
- Modernising Medical Careers (www.mmc.nhs.uk).
- National electronic Library for Health (www.nelh.nhs.uk).
- NHS Professionals (www.nhsprofessionals.nhs.uk).
- Trent Deanery (www.nottingham.ac.uk/mid-trent-deanery).
- West Midlands Deanery (www.wmdeanery.org).

Chapter 4: Career support and career fairs

- *BMJ Careers* (www.bmjcareers.com). There is a 'users' guide' leaflet to accompany this.
- Modernising Medical Careers (www.mmc.nhs.uk).

Chapter 6: Broadening your clinical experience

- Department of Health (www.dh.gov.uk). A home of publications and policies.
- National Institute for Health and Clinical Excellence (www.nice.org.uk). A home of publications and policies.

Chapter 11: What's good about a career in medicine?

- NHS Careers (www.nhscareers.nhs.uk).

Chapter 13: Preparation for future jobs

- (www.careers.lon.ac.uk). Includes an example of a poor résumé and the same information presented well.
- Doctors' Supportline, 38 Harwood Road, London SW6 4PD (0870 765 0001; www.doctorssupportline.org).
- Doctors' Support Network, PO Box 360, Stevenage SG1 9AS (0870 321 0642; www.dsn.org.uk).
- Doctors' Support Network Wales and Southwest, 5 Borage Close, Pontprennaeu, Cardiff CF23 8SJ (0870 321 0642).
- GP recruitment (www.gprecruitment.org.uk). Online application system for GP training.
- Jobscore (www.bmjcareers.com/jobscore). Requires free registration.
- Medical interviews (www.medical-interviews.co.uk). Some practical advice for medical interviews.
- Modernising Medical Careers (www.mmc.nhs.uk). The career advice link contains links to personal accounts of working in different specialties.

Chapter 16: Working abroad

- www.amc.org.au. Australian Medical Council.
- www.australia.org.uk. For visas needed to work in Australia.
- www.dest.gov.au. Australian Government, Department of Education, Science and Training.
- www.ecfmg.org. Educational Commission for Foreign Medical Graduates.
- www.health.gov.au. For information on Australian healthcare.
- www.immi.gov.au. Information on visas and immigration.
- www.medicstravel.com. Information for doctors and nurses planning work and electives in hospitals and medical schools abroad.
- www.usmle.org. Information on the United States Medical Licensing Examination.

Chapter 17: Diverse medical careers

- British Association of Sport and Exercise Medicine (www.basem.co.uk).
- British Institute of Musculoskeletal Medicine (www.bimm.org.uk).
- United Kingdom Association of Doctors in Sport (www.ukadis.org).

Chapter 19: Societies and organisations

- British Medical Association, BMA House, Tavistock Square, London WC1H 9JP (020 738 74499; www.bma.org.uk).
- General Medical Council, Regent's Place, 350 Euston Road, London NW1 3JN (0845 357 3456; www.gmc-uk.org).
- Howden Medical Insurance Services, Howden Insurance Brokers, Bevis Marks House, Bevis Marks, London EC3A 7NE (020 762 33806; www.hmis.co.uk).
- Joint Committee of Higher Medical Training (www.jchmt.org.uk).
- Medical Defence Union (www.the-mdu.com).
- Medical and Dental Defence Union of Scotland, Mackintosh House, 120 Blythswood Street, Glasgow G2 2EA (0141 221 5858; www.mddus.com).
- Medical Insurance Agency, MIA, King's Court, London Road, Stevenage SG1 2GA (01438 739739; www.towergate.co.uk).
- Medical Protection Society, Granary Wharf House, Leeds LS11 5PY (0845 605 4000; www.mps.org.uk).
- Medical Sickness, Wesleyan Assurance Society, Colmore Circus, Birmingham B4 6AR (0808 100 1884; www.medical-sickness.co.uk/).
- Medical Women's Federation, Tavistock House North, Tavistock Square, London WC1H 9HX (020 738 77765; www.medicalwomensfederation.org.uk).
- Medical Women's International Association (www.mwia.net/).
- PasTest, Egerton Court, Parkgate Estate, Knutsford WA16 8DX (01565 752000; www.pastest.co.uk).
- Postgraduate Medical Education and Training Board, PMETB, Hercules House, Hercules Road, London SE1 7DU (020 716 06100; www.pmetb.org.uk).

Chapter 20: Discrimination and how to avoid it

- Abilitynet (www.abilitynet.co.uk).
- Access to Work (www.jobcentreplus.gov.uk/cms.asp?Page=/Home/Customers/HelpForDisabledPeople/AccesstoWork).
- Advisory, Conciliation and Arbitration Service (ACAS) (www.acas.org.uk/).
- Association of Disabled Professionals (www.adp.org.uk).
- BMJ Careers Chronic Illness Matching Scheme (www.bmjcareers.com/chill).
- BMJ Careers Discrimination Matching Scheme (www.bmjcareers.com/discrimination).
- British Medical Association (www.bma.org.uk).
- Citizens Advice Bureau (www.nacab.org.uk/).
- Commission for Racial Equality (www.cre.gov.uk).
- Department of Trade and Industry (www.dti.gov.uk/er/index.htm).
- Disability Discrimination Act (www.disability.gov.uk/dda/).
- Disability Rights Commission (www.drc-gb.org).
- Doctors' Supportline (www.doctorssupportline.org).

- Doctors' Support Network (www.dsn.org.uk).
- Doctors' Support Network Wales and Southwest (0870 321 0642).
- Employment Law (www.compactlaw.co.uk/monster/empf30.html).
- Equal Opportunities Commission (www.eoc.org.uk).
- Gay and Lesbian Association for Doctors and Dentists (GLADD) (www.gladd.org.uk).
- Medical Council on Alcohol (www.medicouncilalcol.demon.co.uk).
- SKILL: National Bureau for Students with Disabilities (www.skill.org.uk).
- Workstep (www.jobcentreplus.gov.uk/cms.asp?Page=/Home/Customers/HelpForDisabledPeople/WORKSTEP).

Appendix 2

Current career interests

Date
What type of career interests you at the moment?
Which areas of future career possibilities do not interest you?

Strengths	Weaknesses
What are your strengths?	What are your weaknesses?

Opportunities	Threats
What opportunities are available to help you pursue your career of interest?	What obstacles to your future career do you face?

What, if anything, can you do to overcome your weaknesses?
What is your ideal work–life balance?
What are your career aspirations?
Looking at the answers to the above, and at the appropriate specialty profile within this book, comment on your suitability to your career of interest.
What expectations, questions or concerns do you have at this stage about your career?
Photocopy this page for your own use

Appendix 3

Using clinical attachments to further career development decisions

Attachment
Date
Which aspects of this attachment did you enjoy?
Which aspects of this attachment did you not enjoy?
What type of experiences were you exposed to?
What did you learn about yourself during this attachment?
What feedback did you receive?
What strengths do you think are required for a career within this specialty?
Which aspects of this attachment would you like to do more of in the future?
Would you consider the area of your attachment for your future career? (State reasons)
Photocopy this page for your own use

Appendix 4

Contact details for the Royal Colleges

- **Academy of Medical Royal Colleges** 1 Wimpole Street, London W1G 0AE (+44 (0)20 740 82244; www.aomrc.org.uk).
- **Royal College of Anaesthetists** 48/49 Russell Square, London WC1B 4JP (+44 (0)20 790 87300; www.rcoa.ac.uk).
- **Royal College of General Practitioners** 14 Princes Gate, Hyde Park, London SW7 1PU (+44 (0)20 758 13232; www.rcgp.org.uk).
- **Royal College of General Practitioners Northern Ireland** Building 4, Ground Floor, Cromac Place, Ormeau Road, Belfast BT7 2JB (+44 (0)289 023 0055; www.rcgp-ni.org.uk).
- **Royal College of General Practitioners Scotland** 25 Queen Street, Edinburgh EH2 1JX (+44 (0)131 260 6800; www.rcgp-scotland.org.uk).
- **Royal College of General Practitioners Wales** Regus House, Falcon Drive, Cardiff Bay, Cardiff CF10 4RU (+44 (0)292 050 4604; www.rcgp.wales.nhs.uk).
- **Royal College of Obstetricians and Gynaecologists** 27 Sussex Place, London NW1 4RG (+44 (0)20 777 26200; www.rcog.org.uk).
- **Royal College of Paediatrics and Child Health** 50 Hallam Street, London W1N 6DE (+44 (0)20 730 75600; www.rcpch.ac.uk).
- **Royal College of Ophthalmologists** 17 Cornwall Terrace, London NW1 4QW (+44 (0)20 793 50702; www.rcophth.ac.uk).
- **Royal College of Pathologists** 2 Carlton House Terrace, London SW1Y 5AF (+44 (0)20 745 16700; www.rcpath.org).
- **Royal College of Physicians** 11 St Andrew's Place, Regent's Park, London NW1 4LE (+44 (0)20 793 51174; www.rcplondon.ac.uk).
- **Royal College of Physicians of Edinburgh** 9 Queen Street, Edinburgh EH2 1JQ (+44 (0)131 225 7324; www.rcpe.ac.uk).
- **Royal College of Physicians and Surgeons of Glasgow** 232–242 St Vincent Street, Glasgow G2 5RJ (+44 (0)141 221 6072; www.rcpsglasg.ac.uk).
- **Royal College of Psychiatrists** 17 Belgrave Square, London SW1X 8PG (+44 (0)20 723 52351; www.rcpsych.ac.uk).
- **Royal College of Psychiatrists Northern Irish Division** Forsyth Business Centre, 2–14 East Bridge Street, Belfast BT1 3MQ (+44 (0)289 092 3763; www.rcpsych.ac.uk/college/division/northernireland.asp).
- **Royal College of Psychiatrists Scottish Division** 12 Queen Street, Edinburgh EH2 1JE (+44 (0)131 220 2915; www.rcpsych.ac.uk/college/division/scot.asp).
- **Royal College of Psychiatrists Welsh Division** Baltic House, Mount Stuart Square, Cardiff CF10 5FH (+44 (0)292 048 9006; www.rcpsych.ac.uk/college/division/welsh.asp).
- **Royal College of Radiologists** 38 Portland Place, London W1N 3DG (+44 (0)20 763 64432; www.rcr.ac.uk).

- **Royal College of Surgeons of England** 25–43 Lincoln's Inn Fields, London WC2A 3PN (+44 (0)20 740 53474; www.rcseng.ac.uk).
- **Royal College of Surgeons of Edinburgh** Nicolson Street, Edinburgh EH8 9DW (+44 (0)131 527 1600; www.rcsed.ac.uk).

Appendix 5

Medical schools in the UK

All contact details correct at the time of print. The medical schools listed below run various medical degrees; to get more detailed information, e-mail addresses and information on each university please visit the websites listed below. The website addresses in brackets are for the medical schools.

- **Aberdeen** – School of Medicine, University of Aberdeen, Polwarth Building, Foresterhill, Aberdeen AB25 2ZD +44 (0)122 455 3015/4975 www.abdn.ac.uk (www.abdn.ac.uk/medicine)
- **Belfast** – Queen's University, Whitla Medical Building, 97 Lisburn Road, Belfast BT9 7BL +44 (0)289 033 5778 www.qub.ac.uk (www.qub.ac.uk/cm)
- **Birmingham** – The University of Birmingham, Edgbaston, Birmingham B15 2TT +44 (0)121 414 6888/3687 www.bham.ac.uk (www.medicine.bham.ac.uk)
- **Brighton** – Brighton and Sussex Medical School, BSMS Teaching Building, University of Sussex, Brighton BN1 9PX +44 (0)127 364 4644 www.bsms.ac.uk (www.bsms.ac.uk)
- **Bristol** – Faculty of Medicine and Dentistry, 69 St Michael's Hill, Bristol BS1 8DZ +44 (0)117 928 7679 www.bristol.ac.uk (www.medici.bris.ac.uk)
- **Cambridge** – University of Cambridge, School of Clinical Medicine, Addenbrooke's Hospital, Hills Road, Cambridge CB2 2SP +44 (0)122 333 6700 www.cam.ac.uk (www.medschl.cam.ac.uk)
- **Cardiff** – University of Wales, School of Medicine Registry, University of Wales College of Medicine, Heath Park, Cardiff CG14 4XN +44 (0)292 074 2027/3436 www.cardiff.ac.uk (www.cardiff.ac.uk/medicine)
- **Dundee** – Faculty of Medicine, Dentistry and Nursing, University of Dundee, Level 10, Ninewells Hospital and Medical School, Dundee DD1 9YS +44 (0)138 263 2763 www.dundee.ac.uk (www.dundee.ac.uk/medical school)
- **Durham** – Stockton, University of Durham, Queen's Campus Stockton, University Boulevard, Stockton-on-Tees TS17 6BH +44 (0)191 334 0048 www.dur.ac.uk (www.dur.ac.uk/phase1.medicine)
- **Edinburgh** – College of Medicine and Veterinary Medicine, The University of Edinburgh, The Queen's Medical Research Institute, 47 Little France Crescent, Edinburgh EH16 4TJ +44 (0)131 242 9300 www.ed.ac.uk (www.mvm.ed.ac.uk)
- **Glasgow** – Faculty of Medicine, Wolfson Medical School Building, University Avenue, University of Glasgow G12 8QQ +44 (0)141 330 5921 www.gla.ac.uk (www.gla.ac.uk/departments/medicineroyal./home.htm)
- **Hull** – The University of Hull, Hull HU6 7RX +44 (0)148 246 4705 (www.hyms.ac.uk)
- **York** – The University of York, Heslington, York YO10 5DD +44 (0)190 432 1969 (www.hyms.ac.uk)

- **Keele** – School of Medicine, Keele University, Keele ST5 5BG +44 (0)178 258 3642/3632 www.keele.ac.uk (www.keele.ac.uk/depts/ms)
- **Leeds** – Faculty of Medicine and Health, Worsley Building, University of Leeds, Leeds LS2 9JT +44 (0)113 343 7194 www.leeds.ac.uk (www.leeds.ac.uk/medicine/index.html)
- **Leicester** – University of Leicester, Medical School, University Road, Leicester LE1 7RH +44 (0)116 252 5281 www.le.ac.uk (www.le.ac.uk/sm/le)
- **Liverpool** – University of Liverpool, Faculty of Medicine, Duncan Building, Daulby Street, Liverpool L69 3GA +44 (0)151 706 4261 www.liv.ac.uk (www.liv.ac.uk/medicine)
- **London** – Barts and The London, Queen Mary University of London, Turner Street, London E1 2AD +44 (0)20 737 77611 www.qmul.ac.uk (www.mds.qmw.ac.uk)
- **London** – King's College, King's College London School of Medicine, First Floor, Hodgkin Building, Guys Campus, London SE1 9RT +44 (0)20 783 65454 www.klc.ac.uk (www.kcl.ac.uk/teares/gktvc)
- **London** – Imperial College, Imperial College School of Medicine, South Kensington Campus, London SW7 2AZ +44 (0)20 759 48800 www.imperial.ac.uk (www1.imperial.ac.uk/medicine/default/html)
- **London** – Royal Free and University College, University College London, Gower Street, London WC1E 6BT +44 (0)20 767 97050 www.ucl.ac.uk (www.ucl.ac.uk/medicalschool)
- **London** – St George's, St George's Hospital Medical School, Cranmer Terrace, London SW17 0RE +44 (0)20 867 29944 www.sgul.ac.uk
- **Manchester** – The University of Manchester, Oxford Road, Manchester M13 9PL +44 (0)161 275 2077 www.manchester.ac.uk (www.medicine.manchester.ac.uk.
- **Newcastle upon Tyne** – University of Newcastle upon Tyne, 10 Kensington Terrace, Newcastle upon Tyne NE1 7RU +44 (0)191 222 5594 www.ncl.ac.uk (www.medical.faculty.ncl.ac.uk)
- **Norwich** – University of East Anglia, School of Medicine, Norwich NR4 7TJ +44 (0)160 345 6161 www.uea.ac.uk (www.med.uea.ac.uk)
- **Nottingham** – Faculty of Medicine and Health Sciences, University of Nottingham Medical School, Queen's Medical Centre, Nottingham NG7 2UH +44 (0)115 970 9379 www.nottingham.ac.uk (www.nottingham.ac.uk/mhs)
- **Oxford** – The Medical Sciences Office, University of Oxford, The John Radcliffe Hospital, Oxford OX3 9DU +44 (0)186 522 1689 www.ox.ac.uk (www.medsci.ox.ac.uk)
- **Peninsula Medical School** – Peninsula Medical School, John Bull Building, Research Way, Plymouth PL6 8BU +44 (0)175 243 7444 www.pms.ac.uk (www.pms.ac.uk/pms)
- **Sheffield** – School of Medicine and Biomedical Sciences, University of Sheffield, Beech Hill Road, Sheffield S10 2RX +44 (0)114 271 3349 www.sheffield.ac.uk (www.shef.ac.uk/medicine)
- **Southampton** – School of Medicine, Southampton General Hospital, Tremona Road, Southampton SO16 6YD +44 (0)238 079 6586 www.soton.ac.uk (www.som.soton.ac.uk)
- **St Andrews** – The University of St Andrews, 79 North Street, St Andrews KY16 9AJ +44 (0)133 446 2150/3502 www.st-and.ac.uk (http://medicine.st-and.ac.uk)

- **Swansea** – University of Wales, School of Medicine, Grove Building, University of Wales Swansea, Singleton Park, Swansea SA2 8PP +44 (0)179 251 3400 www2.swan.ac.uk (www.medicine.swan.ac.uk)
- **Warwick** – Warwick Medical School, The University of Warwick, Coventry CV4 7AL +44 (0)247 652 3523 www.warwick.ac.uk (www2.warwick.ac.uk/fac/med/)

Index